Stahl's Self-Assessment Examination
in Psychiatry
Multiple Choice Questions for Clinicians

Second Edition

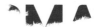

Stahl's Self-Assessment Examination in Psychiatry
Multiple Choice Questions for Clinicians

Second Edition

Stephen M. Stahl
*Adjunct Professor of Psychiatry
at the University of California at San Diego,
San Diego, California, USA and
Honorary Visiting Senior Fellow in Psychiatry
at the University of Cambridge, Cambridge, UK*

Editorial Assistant
Meghan M. Grady

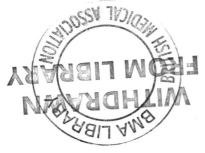

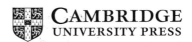

CAMBRIDGE
UNIVERSITY PRESS

CAMBRIDGE
UNIVERSITY PRESS

University Printing House, Cambridge CB2 8BS, United Kingdom

Cambridge University Press is part of the University of Cambridge.

It furthers the University's mission by disseminating knowledge in the pursuit of
education, learning and research at the highest international levels of excellence.

www.cambridge.org
Information on this title: www.cambridge.org/9781316502495

© Neuroscience Education Institute 2016

First published 2012
Second edition 2016

Printed in the United States of America by Sheridan Books, Inc.

A catalog record for this publication is available from the British Library

Library of Congress Cataloging-in-Publication Data

Stahl, Stephen M., 1951–, author.
  Stahl's self-assessment examination in psychiatry : multiple choice questions for
clinicians / Stephen M. Stahl ; editorial assistant, Meghan M. Grady. – Second edition.
    p. ; cm.
  Includes index.
  ISBN 978-1-316-50249-5 (Paperback)
  I. Title.
  [DNLM: 1. Mental Disorders–Examination Questions.   2. Nervous System
Physiological Phenomena–Examination Questions.   3. Psychiatry–methods–
Examination Questions. WM 18.2]
  RC457
  616.890076–dc23   2015024714

ISBN 978-1-316-50249-5 Paperback

CONTENTS

INTRODUCTION/PREFACE

As many readers know, *Essential Psychopharmacology* started in 1996 as a textbook (currently in its fourth edition) on **how psychotropic drugs work** and then expanded to a companion *Prescriber's Guide* in 2005 (currently in its fifth edition) on **how to prescribe psychotropic drugs**. In 2008, a website was added (*stahlonline.org*) with both of these books available online in combination with several more, including an *Illustrated* series of several books covering specialty topics in psychopharmacology. In 2011 a case book was added, called *Case Studies: Stahl's Essential Psychopharmacology* that shows **how to apply the concepts** presented in these previous books **to real patients in a clinical practice setting**. Now comes a comprehensive set of questions and answers that we call *Stahl's Self-Assessment Examination in Psychiatry: Multiple Choice Questions for Clinicians*, designed to be integrated into the suite of our mental health/psychopharmacology books and products in the manner that I will explain here.

Why a question book?

Classically, test questions are used to measure learning, and the questions in this new book can certainly be used in this traditional manner, both by teachers and by students, and especially in combination with the companion textbook in this suite of educational products, *Stahl's Essential Psychopharmacology*. That is, teachers may wish to test student learning following their lectures on these topics by utilizing these questions and answers as part of a final examination. Also, readers not taking a formal course may wish to quiz themselves after studying specific topics in the specific chapters of the textbook. The reader will also note that documentation of the answers to each question in the SAE book refers the reader back to the specific section of the textbook where that answer can be found and explained in great detail; outside references for the answers to the questions in the SAE book are also provided.

Do questions just document learning?

For the modern self-directed learner, questions do much more than just document learning; they can also provide beacons for what needs to be studied and the motivation for doing that even before you read a textbook. Thus, questions are also tools for pre-study self-assessment. If you want to know whether you have already mastered a certain area of psychopharmacology, you can ask yourself these SAE questions BEFORE you review any specific area in the field. Many reading a textbook of psychopharmacology are not novices, but lifelong learners, and are likely to have areas of strength as well as areas of weakness. Getting correct answers will show you that a specific area is already well understood. On the other hand, getting lots of incorrect answers not only informs the self-motivated learner that a specific area needs further study, but can provide the motivation for that learner to fill in the gaps. Failure can be a powerful focuser for what to study and an energizing motivator for why to study.

"Adults don't want answers to questions they have not asked"

The truth of this old saying is that taking a test AFTER study tends to feel like being forced to answer questions that the teacher has asked. However, modern readers with the mind-set of a self-directed learner want to focus on gaps in their knowledge, so looking at these same questions PRIOR to study is a way of asking the questions of yourself and thus owning them and their answers.

What is a "knowledge sandwich?"

Ideally, self-directed learners organize their study as a "knowledge sandwich" of meaty information lying between two slices of questions. The questions in this SAE book can be the first slice of questioning, followed by consuming the "meat" of the subject material in any textbook, including *Stahl's Essential Psychopharmacology*, or if you prefer, from a lecture, course (such as the integrated Neuroscience Education Institute's annual Psychopharmacology Congress), journal article, whatever. At the end of studying, another slice of testing shows whether learning has occurred, and whether performance has improved. You can utilize, for example, the continuing medical education (CME) tests that accompany either *Stahl's Essential Psychopharmacology* (for up to 90 hours of CME credits) or *Case Studies: Stahl's Essential Psychopharmacology* (for up to 67 hours of CME credits) as two options to test yourself after studying and document your learning (available at *neiglobal. com*). The rationale for this instructional design is also discussed in another relative newcomer to our suite of books, *Best Practices in Medical Teaching*, published in 2011. The SAE questions, additional "meaty" content on all the subject areas, plus posttests are also available as the "Master Psychopharmacology Program" at *neiglobal.com* for those who prefer online learning rather than a textbook.

Recertification/maintenance of certification by the American Board of Psychiatry and Neurology (ABPN)

Utilizing SAE questions as the first "slice" of the learning "sandwich" is not just theoretical, but is gaining prominence among expert educators these days, and indeed is now part of the requirements for maintenance of certification (MOC) in a medical specialty in the USA, including by the ABPN, which has accepted the questions in this SAE book not only for ABPN CME requirements but also for their SA/self-assessment activity requirement, a sort of pretest. For those of you familiar with the Case Studies book in our series, you will know that the Case Studies book also incorporates these educational ideas from the recent changes in MOC by the ABPN for those of you interested in recertification in psychiatry. That is, in the Case Studies book, there is not only a pretest self-assessment question at the beginning of every case, and a posttest knowledge-documenting question at the end of every case, but also practice for the first step of the newly required section from MOC called Performance in Practice (Clinical Module), a short analysis at the end of every case, looking back and seeing what could have been done better in retrospect, another sort of posttest.

Is your learning unforgettable?

Finally, and perhaps most importantly, tests prevent forgetting. Thus, the SAE questions here actually create long-term remembering, and do not just document that initial learning has occurred. It is a sorry fact that learning that occurs following one exposure/ reading of material is rapidly forgotten. We have discussed this in the accompanying book in this series *Best Practices in Medical Teaching*. Perhaps 50% of what you learn after a single exposure to new, complex information is forgotten in 3 to 8 days, with some studies suggesting that little or nothing is remembered in 2 months! Exposing yourself to new material over time in bite-sized chunks and encountering the material again at a later time leads to more retention of information than does learning in a large bolus in a single setting, a concept sometimes called interval learning or spaced learning. Research has shown that when the re-exposure is done not as a review of the same material in the same manner, but as a test, retention is much enhanced. This results in the most efficient way of learning because the initial encoding (reading the material or hearing the lecture the first time) is consolidated for long-term retention much more effectively and completely if the re-exposure is in the form of questions. Thus, questions help you remember, and we hope that you utilize this SAE book to maximize the efficiency of your learning to leverage the time you are able to put into your professional development.

How do you use this book?

To use this book, simply look on every right hand page where you will see the question appear with a multiple choice format for the answer. Read the question, answer the question either in your head, on the page, or on another piece of paper. Then, turn the page and on the left hand will appear not only the correct answer, but also an explanation of why the correct answer is correct, why the incorrect answers are incorrect, and references that document the correct answers, both in the companion textbook *Stahl's Essential Psychopharmacology* and elsewhere. The reader will also see at this time what several hundred peers who have already taken this test thought was the correct answer. While taking a test, the examinee is usually curious about how (s)he is doing, how many peers get a question right, and, if the wrong answer was selected, how many peers also selected that answer wrongly. Such information can provide motivation, either as reinforcement for correct answers (yes!) or to drive the reader to understand the correct answer and never to feel the sting of missing that question again (ouch!).

So, it is with the greatest wishes for your successful journey throughout psychiatry and psychopharmacology that I present this question book to you as one of the tools for your professional development, as well as for your fascination, learning, and remembering!

Stephen M. Stahl, MD, PhD

In memory of Daniel X. Freedman, mentor, colleague, and scientific father.

To Cindy, my wife, best friend, and tireless supporter.

To Jennifer and Victoria, my daughters, for their patience and understanding of the demands of authorship.

CME INFORMATION

Release/expiration dates

Released: May 1, 2015

CME credit expires: April 1, 2018. *If this date has passed, please contact NEI for updated information.*

Overview

These case-based questions, divided into 10 core areas of psychiatry, will help you identify areas in which you need further study. Each question is followed by an explanation of the answer choices and a list of references.

Target audience

This activity has been developed for prescribers specializing in psychiatry. There are no prerequisites. All other health care providers interested in psychopharmacology are welcome for advanced study, especially primary care physicians, nurse practitioners, psychologists, and pharmacists.

Statement of need

Mental disorders are highly prevalent and carry substantial burden that can be alleviated through treatment; unfortunately, many patients with mental disorders do not receive treatment or receive suboptimal treatment. There is a documented gap between evidence-based practice guidelines and actual care in clinical practice for patients with mental illnesses. This gap is due at least in part to lack of clinician confidence and knowledge in terms of appropriate usage of the diagnostic and treatment tools available to them.

To help fill these unmet needs, quality improvement efforts need to provide education regarding: (1) diagnostic strategies that can aid in the identification and differential diagnosis of patients with psychiatric illness; (2) effective clinical strategies for monitoring and treating psychiatric patients; (3) new scientific evidence that is most likely to affect clinical practice and neurobiological and pharmacological research; and (4) strategies to optimize functional outcomes for patients with psychiatric illnesses, including strategies to monitor and maximize adherence and working with patients to set and track recovery-oriented goals.

Learning objectives

After completing the entire book, *Stahl's Self-Assessments in Psychiatry: Multiple Choice Questions for Clinicians, second edition*, you should be better able to:

- Diagnose patients presenting with psychiatric symptoms using accepted diagnostic standards and practices

- Implement evidence-based psychiatric treatment strategies that are aligned with the patient's recovery goals

- Integrate recent advances in diagnostic and treatment strategies into clinical practice according to best practice guidelines

Accreditation and credit designation statements

The Neuroscience Education Institute is accredited by the Accreditation Council for Continuing Medical Education (ACCME) to provide continuing medical education for physicians.

The Neuroscience Education Institute designates this enduring material for a maximum of 14.0 *AMA PRA Category 1 Credits* ™. Physicians should claim only the credit commensurate with the extent of their participation in the activity.

The American Society for the Advancement of Pharmacotherapy (ASAP), Division 55 of the American Psychological Association, is approved by the American Psychological Association to sponsor continuing education for psychologists. ASAP maintains responsibility for this program and its content.

The American Society for the Advancement of Pharmacotherapy designates this program for 14.0 CE credits for psychologists.

Nurses: for all of your CNE requirements for recertification, the ANCC will accept *AMA PRA Category 1 Credits*™ from organizations accredited by the ACCME. The content of this activity pertains to pharmacology and is worth 14.0 continuing education hours of pharmacotherapeutics.

Physician Assistants: the NCCPA accepts *AMA PRA Category 1 Credit ™* from organizations accredited by the AMA (providers accredited by the ACCME).

A certificate of participation for completing this activity will also be available.

Please note: the content of this print monograph also exists as an online learning activity under the title "Master Psychopharmacology Program Self-Assessments, 2015–2017 edition". If you received CME credit for that activity, you will not be able to receive credit again for completing this print monograph.

ABPN – Maintenance of certification (MOC)

The American Board of Psychiatry and Neurology (ABPN) has reviewed *Stahl's Self-Assessments in Psychiatry: Multiple Choice Questions for Clinicians, second edition,* and has approved this program as part of a comprehensive lifelong learning and self-assessment program, which is mandated by the American Board of Medical Specialties (ABMS) as a necessary component of maintenance of certification.

More information about ABPN's Maintenance of Certification Program for psychiatry is available at http://www.abpn.com/maintain-certification

Instructions

The chapters of this book can be completed in any order. You are advised to read each question carefully, formulate an answer, and then review the answer/explanation on the following page. The estimated time for completion of the entire activity (including optional posttests and CME evaluations) is 14.0 hours.

Optional posttests with CME credits are available for a fee (waived for NEI Members). For participant ease, each chapter has its own posttest and certificate. NOTE: the book as a whole is considered a single activity and credits earned must be totaled and submitted as such to other organizations. To receive a certificate of CME credit or participation, complete the chapter posttest and evaluation, available only online at **neiglobal.com/CME** (under "Book"). If a score of 70% or more is attained, you will be able to immediately print your certificate. If you have questions, call 888–535–5600, or email customerservice@neiglobal.com.

CME Information

Peer Review

These materials have been peer-reviewed to ensure the scientific accuracy and medical relevance of information presented and its independence from commercial bias. The Neuroscience Education Institute takes responsibility for the content, quality, and scientific integrity of this CME activity.

Disclosures

It is the policy of NEI to ensure balance, independence, objectivity, and scientific rigor in all its educational activities. Therefore, all individuals in a position to influence or control content are required to disclose any financial relationships. Although potential conflicts of interest are identified and resolved prior to the activity being presented, it remains for the participant to determine whether outside interests reflect a possible bias in either the exposition or the conclusions presented.

Disclosed financial relationships with conflicts of interest have been reviewed by the Neuroscience Education Institute CME Advisory Board Chair and resolved.

Authors

Meghan Grady
Director, Content Development, Neuroscience Education Institute, Carlsbad, CA
No financial relationships to disclose.

Debbi Ann Morrissette, PhD
Adjunct Professor, Biological Sciences, Palomar College, San Marcos, CA
Senior Medical Writer, Neuroscience Education Institute, Carlsbad, CA
No financial relationships to disclose.

(also content editor)
Stephen M. Stahl, MD, PhD
Adjunct Professor, Department of Psychiatry, University of California, San Diego School of Medicine, San Diego, CA
Honorary Visiting Senior Fellow, University of Cambridge, UK
Director of Psychopharmacology, California Department of State Hospitals, CA
Grant/Research: Alkermes, Clintara, Forest, Forum, Genomind, Jay-Mac, Jazz, Lilly, Merck, Novartis, Otsuka America, Pamlab, Pfizer, Servier, Shire, Sprout, Sunovion, Sunovion UK, Takeda, Teva, Tonix

Consultant/Advisor: Acadia, BioMarin, Forum/EnVivo, Jazz, Orexigen, Otsuka America, Pamlab, Servier, Shire, Sprout, Taisho, Takeda, Trius

Speakers Bureau: Forum, Servier, Sunovion UK, Takeda

Board Member: BioMarin, Forum/EnVivo, Genomind, Lundbeck, Otsuka America, RCT Logic, Shire

Peer Reviewer

Ronnie Gorman Swift, MD

Professor and Associate Chairman, Department of Psychiatry and Behavioral Sciences, New York Medical College, Valhalla, NY

Chief of Psychiatry and Associate Medical Director, Metropolitan Hospital Center, New York, NY

No financial relationships to disclose.

Disclosure of off-label use

This educational activity may include discussion of unlabeled and/or investigational uses of agents that are not currently labeled for such use by the FDA. Please consult the product prescribing information for full disclosure of labeled uses.

Disclaimer

Participants have an implied responsibility to use the newly acquired information from this activity to enhance patient outcomes and their own professional development. The information presented in this educational activity is not meant to serve as a guideline for patient management. Any procedures, medications, or other courses of diagnosis or treatment discussed or suggested in this educational activity should not be used by clinicians without evaluation of their patients' conditions and possible contraindications or dangers in use, review of any applicable manufacturer's product information, and comparison with recommendations of other authorities. Primary references and full prescribing information should be consulted.

Cultural and linguistic competency

A variety of resources addressing cultural and linguistic competency can be found at this link: http://www.nei.global/cmeregs

Provider

This CME activity is provided by the Neuroscience Education Institute.

CME Information

Additionally provided by the American Society for the Advancement of Pharmacotherapy.

Support

This activity is supported solely by the Neuroscience Education Institute.

1 BASIC NEUROSCIENCE

QUESTION ONE

An excitatory signal is received at the dendrite of a pyramidal glutamate neuron. When the signal is released from the incoming presynaptic dopaminergic axon, it is received as an inhibitory signal. However, this signal is not integrated properly with other incoming signals to that neuron. Which is the most likely site at which the error of integrating this signal with other incoming signals occurred?

A. Dendritic membrane

B. Soma

C. Axonal zone

D. Presynaptic zone

Answer to Question One

The correct answer is B.

Choice	Peer answers
A. Dendritic membrane	14%
B. Soma	64%
C. Axonal zone	10%
D. Presynaptic zone	12%

A Incorrect. Dendritic membrane is the site of signal detection; signal integration does not occur here.

B Correct. Soma is the site that integrates chemical encoding of signal transduction from all incoming signals; improper signal integration is most likely at this site.

C Incorrect. Axonal zone is the site of signal propagation; signal integration does not occur here.

D Incorrect. Presynaptic zone is the site of signal output; signal integration does not occur here.

References

Schatzberg AF, Nemeroff CB. *Textbook of psychopharmacology*, fourth edition. Washington, DC: American Psychiatric Publishing, Inc.; 2009. (Chapter 2)

Stahl SM. *Stahl's essential psychopharmacology*, fourth edition. New York, NY: Cambridge University Press; 2013. (Chapter 1)

Basic neuroscience

QUESTION TWO

A receptor synthesized with an erroneous amino acid sequence is sent via fast anterograde transport to its axonal destination. If you want to find the original site of error, which organelle would you elect to observe?

A. Free polysome

B. Golgi apparatus

C. Mitochondria

D. Rough endoplasmic reticulum

Answer to Question Two

The correct answer is D.

Choice	Peer answers
A. Free polysome	2%
B. Golgi apparatus	14%
C. Mitochondria	16%
D. Rough endoplasmic reticulum	68%

A   Incorrect. Free polysomes, or non–membrane-bound ribosomes, are the site of peripheral protein (e.g., microtubules, neurofilaments) synthesis.

B   Incorrect. Golgi apparatus is the place to which integral proteins are sent for modification after synthesis.

C   Incorrect. Mitochondria, the cell's "powerhouses," are important energy sources to fuel cellular transport but will not reveal underlying causes of errors in protein synthesis.

D   Correct. The rough endoplasmic reticulum, or membrane-bound ribosomes, is the site of integral protein (e.g., receptors, enzymes, ion channels) synthesis; such proteins are destined for membrane insertion and travel via fast transport.

References

Schatzberg AF, Nemeroff CB. *Textbook of psychopharmacology*, fourth edition. Washington, DC: American Psychiatric Publishing, Inc.; 2009. (Chapter 2)

Stahl SM. *Stahl's essential psychopharmacology*, fourth edition. New York, NY: Cambridge University Press; 2013. (Chapter 1)

QUESTION THREE

Which of the following are involved in regulating neurotransmission via excitation–secretion coupling?

A. Voltage-sensitive sodium channels

B. Voltage-sensitive calcium channels

C. Both A and B

D. Neither A nor B

Answer to Question Three

The correct answer is C.

Choice	Peer answers
A. Voltage-sensitive sodium channels	14%
B. Voltage-sensitive calcium channels	13%
C. Both A and B	67%
D. Neither A nor B	7%

A Partially correct.

B Partially correct.

C Correct. Propagation of an action potential to the axon terminal is mediated by voltage-sensitive sodium channels. Influx of sodium through voltage-sensitive sodium channels at the axon terminal leads to opening of voltage-sensitive calcium channels, also at the axon terminal. Influx of calcium through the open voltage-sensitive calcium channels leads to docking of synaptic vesicles and secretion of neurotransmitter into the synapse.

D Incorrect.

References
Stahl SM. *Stahl's essential psychopharmacology*, fourth edition. New York, NY: Cambridge University Press; 2013. (Chapter 3)

Basic neuroscience

QUESTION FOUR

Agonists cause ligand-gated ion channels to:

A. Open wider

B. Open for longer duration of time

C. Open more frequently

D. A and B

E. A and C

Answer to Question Four

The correct answer is C.

Choice	Peer answers
A. Open wider	5%
B. Open for longer duration of time	13%
C. Open more frequently	36%
D. A and B	24%
E. A and C	23%

A Incorrect. Agonists do not cause ligand-gated receptors to open wider.

B Incorrect. Agonists do not cause ligand-gated receptors to open for longer durations of time.

C Correct. Agonists cause ligand-gated ion channels to open more frequently.

D Incorrect.

E Incorrect.

References

Stahl SM. *Stahl's essential psychopharmacology*, fourth edition. New York, NY: Cambridge University Press; 2013. (Chapter 3)

QUESTION FIVE

Presynaptic reuptake transporters are a major method of inactivation for which of the following?

A. Serotonin

B. Serotonin and GABA

C. Serotonin, GABA, and histamine

D. Serotonin, GABA, histamine, and neuropeptides

Answer to Question Five

The correct answer is B.

Choice	Peer answers
A. Serotonin	36%
B. Serotonin and GABA	38%
C. Serotonin, GABA, and histamine	11%
D. Serotonin, GABA, histamine, and neuropeptides	15%

A Partially correct.

B Correct. Both monoamines such as serotonin and amino acid neuro-transmitters such as GABA are inactivated primarily via presynaptic transporters.

C Incorrect. Histamine does not have a known presynaptic reuptake transporter and is instead inactivated via enzymatic degradation.

D Incorrect. Histamine and neuropeptides do not have known pre-synaptic reuptake transporters. Histamine is inactivated enzymatically and neuropeptides are inactivated by diffusion, sequestration, and enzymatic destruction.

References

Stahl SM. *Stahl's essential psychopharmacology*, fourth edition. New York, NY: Cambridge University Press; 2013. (Chapter 2)

QUESTION SIX

A neuron is infected with a toxin and causes a rather sudden inflammatory reaction. You detect a high concentration of cytokines in the surrounding area. Which process has taken place?

A. Necrosis

B. Synaptogenesis

C. Excitotoxicity

D. Apoptosis

E. Neurogenesis

Basic neuroscience

Answer to Question Six

The correct answer is A.

Choice	Peer answers
A. Necrosis	39%
B. Synaptogenesis	0%
C. Excitotoxicity	27%
D. Apoptosis	31%
E. Neurogenesis	4%

A Correct. Necrosis is the neural selection process in which a cell is poisoned, suffocated, or otherwise destroyed by a toxin after which the cell explodes and causes an inflammatory reaction.

B Incorrect. Synaptogenesis is the process of forming synapses.

C Incorrect. Excitotoxicity is a process of synaptic damage from "over-excitation," excessive amounts of which can result in cell death.

D Incorrect. Apoptosis is triggered by a cell's own genetic machinery, causing the cell to just "fade away." The more caustic inflammatory response from cell death is associated with the neural selection process of necrosis. Cells that commit suicide (apoptosis) die in a more benign manner than when they are the victims of homicide (necrosis).

E Incorrect. Neurogenesis is the process of forming neurons.

References

Schatzberg AF, Nemeroff CB. *Textbook of psychopharmacology*, fourth edition. Washington, DC: American Psychiatric Publishing, Inc.; 2009. (Chapter 1)

Stahl SM. *Stahl's essential psychopharmacology*, fourth edition. New York, NY: Cambridge University Press; 2013. (Chapter 1)

QUESTION SEVEN

Communication between human CNS neurons at synapses is:

A. Chemical

B. Electrical

C. Both A and B

D. Neither A nor B

Answer to Question Seven

The correct answer is A.

Choice	Peer answers
A. Chemical	61%
B. Electrical	0%
C. Both A and B	39%
D. Neither A nor B	0%

A Correct. The communication between neurons at synapses is mediated by neurotransmitter molecules and is therefore chemical.

B Incorrect. Although electrical communication occurs within neurons during the propagation of an action potential, communication at synapses is chemical.

C Incorrect.

D Incorrect.

References
Stahl SM. *Stahl's essential psychopharmacology*, fourth edition. New York, NY: Cambridge University Press; 2013. (Chapter 1)

QUESTION EIGHT

A serotonin molecule binds to a 5HT2A receptor causing electrical impulses to be sent down a GABA neuron's axon terminal, eventually releasing GABA to the $GABA_A$ receptor of its postsynaptic neuron. Which type of neurotransmission does this describe?

A. Classic synaptic neurotransmission

B. Retrograde neurotransmission

C. Volume neurotransmission

D. Signal transduction cascade

Answer to Question Eight

The correct answer is A.

Choice	Peer answers
A. Classic synaptic neurotransmission	76%
B. Retrograde neurotransmission	1%
C. Volume neurotransmission	0%
D. Signal transduction cascade	23%

A Correct. Classic synaptic neurotransmission is the most common and well-known process of neurotransmission. It involves the anterograde transduction of a chemical signal to electrical impulses and back to chemical signals for the next neuron.

B Incorrect. Retrograde neurotransmission is the "reverse" neurotransmission process in which a postsynaptic neuron communicates with a presynaptic neuron.

C Incorrect. Volume neurotransmission is the process of neurotransmission without a synapse, which is also called non-synaptic diffusion.

D Incorrect. Signal transduction cascade is the larger process of neurocommunication that involves long strings of chemical and ionic signals.

References

Schatzberg AF, Nemeroff CB. *Textbook of psychopharmacology*, fourth edition. Washington, DC: American Psychiatric Publishing, Inc.; 2009. (Chapters 1, 4)

Stahl SM. *Stahl's essential psychopharmacology*, fourth edition. New York, NY: Cambridge University Press; 2013. (Chapter 1)

QUESTION NINE

A receptor with four-transmembrane regions changes conformation as GABA binds. Which system is this process describing?

A. Presynaptic transporter

B. Ligand-gated ion channel

C. Voltage-sensitive ion channel

Answer to Question Nine

The correct answer is B.

Choice	Peer answers
A. Presynaptic transporter	4%
B. Ligand-gated ion channel	89%
C. Voltage-sensitive ion channel	7%

A Incorrect. Presynaptic transporters are twelve-transmembrane region transporters that bind to neurotransmitters to transport them across the presynaptic membrane.

B Correct. Ligand-gated ion channels are four-transmembrane region ion channels that open and close under instruction from bound neurotransmitters.

C Incorrect. Voltage-sensitive ion channels are six-transmembrane region ion channels that open and close under instruction from charges or voltages as determined by ion flow.

References

Schatzberg AF, Nemeroff CB. *Textbook of psychopharmacology*, fourth edition. Washington, DC: American Psychiatric Publishing, Inc.; 2009. (Chapter 1)

Stahl SM. *Stahl's essential psychopharmacology*, fourth edition. New York, NY: Cambridge University Press; 2013. (Chapter 3)

Basic neuroscience

QUESTION TEN

The direct role of transcription factors is to:

A. Cause neurotransmitter release

B. Influence gene expression

C. Synthesize enzymes

D. Trigger signal transduction cascades

Answer to Question Ten

The correct answer is B.

Choice	Peer answers
A. Cause neurotransmitter release	1%
B. Influence gene expression	82%
C. Synthesize enzymes	14%
D. Trigger signal transduction cascades	2%

A   Incorrect. Transcription factors do not directly cause neurotransmitter release.

B   Correct. Transcription factors are proteins that bind to promoter sequences of DNA to turn gene expression on and off.

C   Incorrect. Transcription factors do not directly cause enzyme synthesis.

D   Incorrect. Transcription factors do not directly trigger signal transduction cascades.

References
Stahl SM. *Stahl's essential psychopharmacology*, fourth edition. New York, NY: Cambridge University Press; 2013. (Chapter 1)

QUESTION ELEVEN

Which of the following is the most likely impetus for upregulation of D2 receptors on a striatal dopamine neuron?

A. A bound receptor is taken out of circulation

B. A new receptor is bound and put to use

C. A D2 antagonist persistently binds to the receptor

D. A D2 agonist persistently binds to the receptor

Answer to Question Eleven

The correct answer is C.

Choice	Peer answers
A. A bound receptor is taken out of circulation	1%
B. A new receptor is bound and put to use	1%
C. A D2 antagonist persistently binds to the receptor	67%
D. A D2 agonist persistently binds to the receptor	30%

A Incorrect. A bound receptor is usually taken out of circulation when the neuron wants to decrease, not increase, the number of receptors.

B Incorrect. A new receptor being bound and put to use is a result, not an impetus, of upregulation.

C Correct. Antagonists can oppose neurotransmitter actions, potentially signaling the neuron to upregulate synthesis of that receptor type.

D Incorrect. Agonists can mimic neurotransmitter actions, potentially signaling the neuron to downregulate synthesis of that receptor type.

References

Schatzberg AF, Nemeroff CB. *Textbook of psychopharmacology*, fourth edition. Washington, DC: American Psychiatric Publishing, Inc.; 2009. (Chapters 1, 4)

Stahl SM. *Stahl's essential psychopharmacology*, fourth edition. New York, NY: Cambridge University Press; 2013. (Chapters 3, 5)

Basic neuroscience

QUESTION TWELVE

What is the correct order and direction of ion flow into and out of a neuron experiencing an action potential?

A. $Na+$ in, $K+$ out, $Ca2+$ in

B. $Ca2+$ in, $K+$ out, $Na+$ in

C. $K+$ in, $Na+$ in, $Ca2+$ in

D. $Na+$ in, $Ca2+$ in, $K+$ out

E. $Ca2+$ in, $Na+$ out, $K+$ out

F. $K+$ in, $Ca2+$ in, $Na+$ out

Answer to Question Twelve

The correct answer is D.

Choice	Peer answers
A. Na+ in, K+ out, Ca2+ in	39%
B. Ca2+ in, K+ out, Na+ in	5%
C. K+ in, Na+ in, Ca2+ in	0%
D. Na+ in, Ca2+ in, K+ out	49%
E. Ca2+ in, Na+ out, K+ out	4%
F. K+ in, Ca2+ in, Na+ out	4%

A, B, C, E, and F Incorrect.

D Correct. Sodium enters the cell followed by an influx of calcium; potassium exits the neuron at the end of the action potential, restoring the baseline electrical charge in the cell.

References

Schatzberg AF, Nemeroff CB. *Textbook of psychopharmacology*, fourth edition. Washington, DC: American Psychiatric Publishing, Inc.; 2009. (Chapter 1)

Stahl SM. *Stahl's essential psychopharmacology*, fourth edition. New York, NY: Cambridge University Press; 2013. (Chapter 3)

QUESTION THIRTEEN

What is epigenetics?

A. Acquired trait coded for by a change in DNA sequence

B. Acquired trait not coded for by a change in DNA sequence

C. Heritable trait coded for by a change in DNA sequence

D. Heritable trait not coded for by a change in DNA sequence

Answer to Question Thirteen

The correct answer is D.

Choice	Peer answers
A. Acquired trait coded for by a change in DNA sequence	27%
B. Acquired trait not coded for by a change in DNA sequence	11%
C. Heritable trait coded for by a change in DNA sequence	22%
D. Heritable trait not coded for by a change in DNA sequence	41%

D Correct. Genetics is the sequence of DNA that is inherited. Epigenetics is a parallel process that determines whether a given gene (i.e., a sequence of DNA coding for transcription) is expressed into its RNA or is silenced. Thus, epigenetics is a heritable phenotype not coded for by a change in DNA sequence. A good example of epigenetics is cell differentiation. Epigenetic molecular switches turn genes on and off by modifying the structure of chromatin in the cell nucleus. Chromatin is an octet of proteins called histones around which your DNA is wrapped. DNA contains genes as well as promoters that tell genes when to make RNA, which can then go on to make proteins. To silence genes, histones or gene promoter DNA sequences can be methylated. Methylation is often followed by another chemical process called deacetylation, which occurs at histones and inactivates nearby genes. To activate genes, the reverse is done: histones and genes are demethylated and histones are acetylated. All of these processes are regulated by numerous enzymes: methylation is also regulated by the availability of methyl donors.

A, B, and C Incorrect.

References

Stahl SM. Fooling mother nature: epigenetics and novel treatments for psychiatric disorders. *CNS Spectr* 2010;**15**(6):220–7.

Stahl SM. *Stahl's essential psychopharmacology*, fourth edition. New York, NY: Cambridge University Press; 2013. (Chapter 1)

Basic neuroscience

QUESTION FOURTEEN

N–methyl–D–aspartate (NMDA) receptors are activated by:

A. Glutamate

B. Glycine

C. Depolarization

D. Glutamate and glycine

E. Glutamate and depolarization

F. Glycine and depolarization

G. Glutamate, glycine, and depolarization

Answer to Question Fourteen

The correct answer is G.

Choice	Peer answers
A. Glutamate	27%
B. Glycine	1%
C. Depolarization	0%
D. Glutamate and glycine	23%
E. Glutamate and depolarization	11%
F. Glycine and depolarization	0%
G. Glutamate, glycine, and depolarization	39%

G Correct. N–methyl–D–aspartate (NMDA) receptors are ligand-gated ion channels that regulate excitatory postsynaptic neurotransmission triggered by glutamate. In the resting state, NMDA receptors are blocked by magnesium, which plugs the calcium channel. Opening of NMDA glutamate receptors requires the presence of both glutamate and glycine, each of which bind to a different site on the receptor. When magnesium is also bound and the membrane is not depolarized, it prevents the effects of glutamate and glycine and thus does not allow the ion channel to open. In order for the channel to open and permit calcium entry, depolarization must remove magnesium while both glutamate and glycine are bound to their sites.

A through F – Incorrect.

References
Stahl SM. *Stahl's essential psychopharmacology*, fourth edition. New York, NY: Cambridge University Press; 2013. (Chapter 4)

QUESTION FIFTEEN

Neurogenesis has recently been discovered to occur in adults:

A. Only in the dentate gyrus of the hippocampus

B. In the dentate gyrus of the hippocampus and in the olfactory bulb

C. In the dentate gyrus of the hippocampus, in the olfactory bulb, and in the lateral nucleus of the amygdala

D. Throughout the brain

E. Adult neurogenesis does not occur

Answer to Question Fifteen

The correct answer is B.

Choice	Peer answers
A. Only in the dentate gyrus of the hippocampus	6%
B. In the dentate gyrus of the hippocampus and in the olfactory bulb	31%
C. In the dentate gyrus of the hippocampus, in the olfactory bulb, and in the lateral nucleus of the amygdala	20%
D. Throughout the brain	41%
E. Adult neurogenesis does not occur	1%

A Incorrect. Although adult neurogenesis does occur in the dentate gyrus, this is not the only brain region where adult neurogenesis occurs.

B Correct. Adult neurogenesis occurs in both the dentate gyrus of the hippocampus and in the olfactory bulb.

C Incorrect. Although adult neurogenesis occurs in both the dentate gyrus and the olfactory bulb, there is no evidence that adult neurogenesis occurs in the lateral nucleus of the amygdala.

D Incorrect. Adult neurogenesis occurs only in the dentate gyrus and in the olfactory bulb.

E Incorrect.

References
Hagg T. Molecular regulation of adult CNS neurogenesis: an integrated view. *Trends Neurosci* 2005;**28**(11):589–95.

Ming GL, Song H. Adult neurogenesis in the mammalian brain: significant answers and significant questions. *Neuron* 2011;**70**(4):687–702.

QUESTION SIXTEEN

In a G protein-linked signal transduction cascade, the second messenger can be synthesized:

A. In the postsynaptic neuron

B. In the synaptic cleft

C. A and B

D. Neither A nor B

Answer to Question Sixteen

The correct answer is A.

Choice	Peer answers
A. In the postsynaptic neuron	66%
B. In the synaptic cleft	5%
C. A and B	18%
D. Neither A nor B	11%

A Correct. Inside the postsynaptic neuron, an activated ligand-gated receptor binds to a G protein. The G protein changes shape so it can bind to an enzyme. The enzyme then synthesizes a second messenger.

B Incorrect. The first messenger binds to a receptor outside of the postsynaptic neuron, initiating a signal transduction cascade. However, the synthesis of the second messenger takes place within the postsynaptic cell.

C Incorrect.

D Incorrect.

References

Stahl SM. *Stahl's essential psychopharmacology*, fourth edition. New York, NY: Cambridge University Press; 2013. (Chapter 2)

Chapter peer comparison

For the Basic neuroscience section, the correct answer was selected 57% of the time.

2 PSYCHOSIS AND SCHIZOPHRENIA AND ANTIPSYCHOTICS

QUESTION ONE

A 24-year-old male initially presents with acute auditory hallucinations and is treated with medication. Four days later he arrives at your office for evaluation. You observe that he is neatly dressed, avoids eye contact, and gives very short answers to your initial questions. Which of the following questions would be most beneficial for determining his degree of negative symptoms?

A. How often have you visited with friends in the past week?

B. Have the voices you've heard persisted or returned?

C. Have you ever thought about hurting yourself or someone else?

D. In the past week have you had difficulty concentrating?

Answer to Question One

The correct answer is A.

Choice	Peer answers
A. How often have you visited with friends in the past week?	86%
B. Have the voices you've heard persisted or returned?	3%
C. Have you ever thought about hurting yourself or someone else?	6%
D. In the past week have you had difficulty concentrating?	6%

A Correct. How often have you visited with friends in the past week: This is a useful question when assessing for negative symptoms, as an important component of negative symptoms is reduced social drive.

B Incorrect. Have the voices you've heard persisted or returned: Although this question is useful for determining the presence of positive symptoms, it is not applicable to assessment of negative symptoms.

C Incorrect. Have you ever thought about hurting yourself or someone else: This question can help assess for risk of suicide as well as any possible aggression risk, but these are not part of the negative symptom domain.

D Incorrect. In the past week have you had difficulty concentrating: This question is applicable to assessment for cognitive symptoms, but not for negative symptoms.

References
Schatzberg AF, Nemeroff CB. *Textbook of psychopharmacology*, fourth edition. Washington, DC: American Psychiatric Publishing, Inc.; 2009. (Chapter 55)

Stahl SM. *Stahl's essential psychopharmacology*, fourth edition. New York, NY: Cambridge University Press; 2013. (Chapter 4)

Stahl SM, Buckley PF. Negative symptoms of schizophrenia: a problem that will not go away. *Acta Psychiatr Scand* 2007;**15**:4–11.

QUESTION TWO

A 22-year-old man with a history of cognitive and social delay has just been diagnosed with schizophrenia. In early elementary school his language development was normal but he had difficulty reading and was diagnosed with a learning disability. He had increased academic difficulty beginning in high school but did graduate and began working at a supermarket. However, he began to exhibit difficulty functioning, including losing things, trouble following simple directions at work, disorganization, and deterioration in communication. These impairments led to his dismissal from his job; 6 months later he experienced a psychotic episode and was diagnosed with schizophrenia. What pattern of cognitive functioning would you expect for this patient over the long-term course of his illness?

A. Progressive decline in cognitive functioning beyond what is expected with normal aging, with severity of cognitive symptoms independent of psychotic symptom status

B. Progressive decline in cognitive functioning beyond what is expected with normal aging, with severity of cognitive symptoms fluctuating with psychotic symptom status

C. No further decline in cognitive functioning beyond what is expected with normal aging, with severity of cognitive symptoms independent of psychotic symptom status

D. No further decline in cognitive functioning beyond what is expected with normal aging, with severity of cognitive symptoms fluctuating with psychotic symptom status

Answer to Question Two

The correct answer is C.

Choice	Peer answers
A. Progressive decline in cognitive functioning beyond what is expected with normal aging, with severity of cognitive symptoms independent of psychotic symptom status	27%
B. Progressive decline in cognitive functioning beyond what is expected with normal aging, with severity of cognitive symptoms fluctuating with psychotic symptom status	35%
C. No further decline in cognitive functioning beyond what is expected with normal aging, with severity of cognitive symptoms independent of psychotic symptom status	27%
D. No further decline in cognitive functioning beyond what is expected with normal aging, with severity of cognitive symptoms fluctuating with psychotic symptom status	11%

C Correct. Like most individuals who ultimately develop schizophrenia, this man had cognitive impairment from an early age and showed substantial further decline in cognitive functioning during late adolescence (during the prodrome phase). However, a large body of research shows that after disorder onset cognitive deficits generally remain stable over the course of the disorder, and do not worsen beyond that expected with normal aging. Additionally, cognitive impairment in schizophrenia does not seem to be correlated with psychotic symptoms.

A, B, and D Incorrect.

References

Schatzberg AF, Nemeroff CB. *Textbook of psychopharmacology*, fourth edition. Washington, DC: American Psychiatric Publishing, Inc.; 2009. (Chapter 55)

Stahl SM. *Stahl's essential psychopharmacology*, fourth edition. New York, NY: Cambridge University Press; 2013. (Chapter 4)

Stahl SM, Buckley PF. Negative symptoms of schizophrenia: a problem that will not go away. *Acta Psychiatr Scand* 2007;**15**:4–11.

QUESTION THREE

A 24-year-old woman is hospitalized after an altercation in which she screamed at and attacked her neighbor when he knocked on her door. Her mother reports that she has been increasingly erratic recently, with emotional outbursts and impulsive behavior. Which of the following brain regions is most likely associated with these symptoms?

A. Dorsolateral prefrontal cortex

B. Nucleus accumbens

C. Orbital frontal cortex

D. Substantia nigra

Answer to Question Three

The correct answer is C.

Choice	Peer answers
A. Dorsolateral prefrontal cortex	36%
B. Nucleus accumbens	6%
C. Orbital frontal cortex	57%
D. Substantia nigra	1%

A Incorrect. Dorsolateral prefrontal cortex: This brain region is hypothetically associated with cognition and executive functioning, not with aggression.

B Incorrect. Nucleus accumbens: This brain region is hypothetically associated with positive symptoms such as delusions and hallucinations. Although aggressive symptoms, such as those exhibited by this patient, often occur in conjunction with positive symptoms, they may not be localized to the nucleus accumbens.

C Correct. Orbital frontal cortex: Aggressive symptoms such as those exhibited by this patient are hypothetically associated with impairment in impulse control, which is largely regulated by the orbital frontal cortex.

D Incorrect. Substantia nigra: This region in the brainstem houses dopaminergic cell bodies that project to the striatum. The substantia nigra is not particularly linked to aggression.

References

Schatzberg AF, Nemeroff CB. *Textbook of psychopharmacology*, fourth edition. Washington, DC: American Psychiatric Publishing, Inc.; 2009. (Chapter 46)

Stahl SM. *Stahl's essential psychopharmacology*, fourth edition. New York, NY: Cambridge University Press; 2013. (Chapter 4)

Stahl SM, Mignon L. *Stahl's illustrated antipsychotics*, second edition. Carlsbad, CA: NEI Press; 2009. (Chapter 1)

QUESTION FOUR

A 44-year-old male with schizophrenia has been taking an anti-psychotic medication since initial diagnosis 12 years ago. He has recently begun experiencing difficulty with fluid movement of his arms as well as involuntary facial grimaces. Which of the following likely underlies these symptoms?

A. Upregulation of serotonin 2A receptors

B. Downregulation of serotonin 2A receptors

C. Upregulation of dopamine 2 receptors

D. Downregulation of dopamine 2 receptors

Answer to Question Four

The correct answer is C.

Choice	Peer answers
A. Upregulation of serotonin 2A receptors	3%
B. Downregulation of serotonin 2A receptors	2%
C. Upregulation of dopamine 2 receptors	69%
D. Downregulation of dopamine 2 receptors	26%

The patient's emerging motor symptoms are indicative of possible development of tardive dyskinesia, a condition characterized by facial and tongue movements as well as by jerky limb movements.

A and B Incorrect. Tardive dyskinesia is not associated with changes in serotonin 2A receptors.

C Correct. Tardive dyskinesia is associated with upregulation of dopamine 2 receptors. This upregulation can occur following long-term blockade of dopamine 2 receptors such as may occur with long-term antipsychotic treatment, particularly conventional antipsychotic treatment.

D Incorrect. Tardive dyskinesia is associated with upregulation, not downregulation, of dopamine 2 receptors.

References

Schatzberg AF, Nemeroff CB. *Textbook of psychopharmacology*, fourth edition. Washington, DC: American Psychiatric Publishing, Inc.; 2009. (Chapter 27)

Stahl SM. *Stahl's essential psychopharmacology*, fourth edition. New York, NY: Cambridge University Press; 2013. (Chapter 5)

Stahl SM, Mignon L. *Stahl's illustrated antipsychotics*, second edition. Carlsbad, CA: NEI Press; 2009. (Chapter 2)

QUESTION FIVE

Based on thorough evaluation of a patient and his history, his care provider intends to begin treatment with a conventional antipsychotic but has not selected a particular agent yet. Which of the following is most true about conventional antipsychotics?

A. They are very similar in therapeutic profile but differ in side-effect profile

B. They are very similar in both therapeutic and side-effect profile

C. They differ in therapeutic profile but are similar in side-effect profile

D. They differ in both therapeutic and side-effect profile

Answer to Question Five

The correct answer is A.

Choice	Peer answers
A. They are very similar in therapeutic profile but differ in side-effect profile	84%
B. They are very similar in both therapeutic and side-effect profile	11%
C. They differ in therapeutic profile but are similar in side-effect profile	2%
D. They differ in both therapeutic and side-effect profile	3%

A Correct. Although individual effects may vary from patient to patient, in general conventional antipsychotics share the same primary mechanism of action and do not differ much in their therapeutic profiles. There are, however, differences in secondary properties, such as degree of muscarinic, histaminergic, and/or alpha adrenergic receptor antagonism, which can lead to different side-effect profiles.

B, C, and D Incorrect.

References

Schatzberg AF, Nemeroff CB. *Textbook of psychopharmacology*, fourth edition. Washington, DC: American Psychiatric Publishing, Inc.; 2009. (Chapter 27)

Stahl SM. *Essential psychopharmacology, the prescriber's guide*, fifth edition. New York, NY: Cambridge University Press; 2014.

Stahl SM. *Stahl's essential psychopharmacology*, fourth edition. New York, NY: Cambridge University Press; 2013. (Chapter 5)

QUESTION SIX

A 34-year-old male recently began experiencing breast secretions while receiving perphenazine. After switching to quetiapine the secretions ceased. Which of the following is the most likely pharmacological explanation for the resolution of this side effect?

A. Dopamine 2 antagonism

B. Serotonin 2A antagonism

C. Serotonin 2C antagonism

D. Histamine 1 antagonism

Psychosis and schizophrenia and antipsychotics

Answer to Question Six

The correct answer is B.

Choice	Peer answers
A. Dopamine 2 antagonism	44%
B. Serotonin 2A antagonism	48%
C. Serotonin 2C antagonism	6%
D. Histamine 1 antagonism	2%

A Incorrect. Stimulation of D2 receptors inhibits prolactin release; thus a dopamine 2 antagonist such as perphenazine could increase prolactin release and potentially lead to breast secretions.

B Correct. Stimulation of serotonin 2A receptors stimulates prolactin release. Since they have opposing effects on prolactin, adding serotonin 2A antagonism to dopamine 2 antagonism results in a neutral effect on prolactin and may relieve breast secretions caused by dopamine 2 antagonism alone.

C and D Incorrect. Although quetiapine is an antagonist at serotonin 2C and histamine 1 receptors, both of which are associated with some side effects, neither receptor type has an established role in prolactin elevation.

References

Schatzberg AF, Nemeroff CB. *Textbook of psychopharmacology*, fourth edition. Washington, DC: American Psychiatric Publishing, Inc.; 2009. (Chapters 28–33)

Stahl SM. *Stahl's essential psychopharmacology*, fourth edition. New York, NY: Cambridge University Press; 2013. (Chapter 5)

Stahl SM, Mignon L. *Stahl's illustrated antipsychotics*, second edition. Carlsbad, CA: NEI Press; 2009. (Chapter 2)

QUESTION SEVEN

A 37-year-old woman with schizophrenia has failed to respond to two sequential adequate trials of antipsychotic monotherapy (first olanzapine, then aripiprazole). Which of the following are evidence-based treatment strategies for a patient in this situation?

A. High dose of her current monotherapy (aripiprazole)

B. Augmentation of her current monotherapy with another atypical antipsychotic

C. Switch to clozapine

D. A and C

E. A, B, and C

Answer to Question Seven

The correct answer is C.

Choice	Peer answers
A. High dose of her current monotherapy (aripiprazole)	0%
B. Augmentation of her current monotherapy with another atypical antipsychotic	7%
C. Switch to clozapine	67%
D. A and C	20%
E. A, B, and C	7%

A Incorrect. Controlled studies for high doses of antipsychotics are quite limited. In particular, the limited data that exist for aripiprazole suggest that it is not usually more effective at doses above the usual recommended range (i.e., 15–30 mg/day for psychosis). Before resorting to high-dose monotherapy, evidence-based strategies for treatment resistance should be exhausted, including the use of clozapine.

B Incorrect. There is limited evidence to support the superior efficacy of combining antipsychotics vs. switching to clozapine or another monotherapy. Controlled studies are limited and review of the evidence that does exist (clinical trials and case reports) has not led to recommendations for antipsychotic polypharmacy in routine clinical practice.

C Correct. After failure of two sequential adequate trials of antipsychotic monotherapy, the recommended and evidence-based treatment strategy is to switch to clozapine.

D Incorrect (A and C).

E Incorrect (A, B, and C).

References

Pandurangi AK, Dalkilic A. Polypharmacy with second-generation antipsychotics: a review of evidence. *J Psychiatr Pract* 2008;**14**:345.

Royal College of Psychiatrists. CR138. Consensus Statement on High-Dose Antipsychotic Medication. 2006. http://www.rcpsych.ac.uk/files/pdfversion/CR138.pdf.

Stahl SM. *Essential psychopharmacology, the prescriber's guide*, fifth edition. New York, NY: Cambridge University Press; 2014.

QUESTION EIGHT

A 24-year-old patient with schizophrenia who has prominent cognitive symptoms and social impairment is being evaluated for treatment. Her care provider is considering initiating ziprasidone, quetiapine, or aripiprazole, all of which share the property of serotonin 1A agonism. This receptor binding property is expected to have clinical effects in schizophrenia most similar to:

A. Serotonin 2A antagonism

B. Dopamine 2 antagonism

C. Histamine 1 antagonism

D. Serotonin transporter blockade

Answer to Question Eight

The correct answer is A.

Choice	Peer answers
A. Serotonin 2A antagonism	44%
B. Dopamine 2 antagonism	29%
C. Histamine 1 antagonism	3%
D. Serotonin transporter blockade	24%

A Correct. Serotonin 2A antagonism: Serotonin 1A partial agonism has similar net effects to serotonin 2A antagonism. That is, it enhances dopamine release and thus may theoretically improve extrapyramidal side effects, hyperprolactinemia, and cognitive and negative symptoms.

B Incorrect. Dopamine 2 antagonism: Serotonin 1A partial agonism enhances dopamine release, whereas dopamine 2 antagonism prevents dopaminergic stimulation of D2 receptors. Thus these mechanisms would not lead to similar clinical effects.

C Incorrect. Histamine 1 antagonism: Serotonin 1A partial agonism and histamine 1 antagonism do not lead to similar clinical effects.

D Incorrect. Serotonin transporter blockade: Serotonin 1A partial agonism and serotonin transporter blockade do not lead to similar clinical effects.

References

Schatzberg AF, Nemeroff CB. *Textbook of psychopharmacology*, fourth edition. Washington, DC: American Psychiatric Publishing, Inc.; 2009. (Chapters 28–33)

Stahl SM. *Essential psychopharmacology, the prescriber's guide*, fifth edition. New York, NY: Cambridge University Press; 2014.

Stahl SM. *Stahl's essential psychopharmacology*, fourth edition. New York, NY: Cambridge University Press; 2013. (Chapter 5)

Stahl SM, Mignon L. *Stahl's illustrated antipsychotics*, second edition. Carlsbad, CA: NEI Press; 2009. (Chapter 4)

QUESTION NINE

A 24-year-old man has just been diagnosed with schizophrenia. His clinician elects to prescribe iloperidone and begins treatment according to the dosing schedule in the label. What is the rationale for the slow dosing schedule with iloperidone?

A. Minimize agitation

B. Minimize sedation

C. Prevent orthostatic hypotension

D. Prevent gastrointestinal upset

Answer to Question Nine

The correct answer is C.

Choice	Peer answers
A. Minimize agitation	9%
B. Minimize sedation	4%
C. Prevent orthostatic hypotension	88%
D. Prevent gastrointestinal upset	0%

A Incorrect (minimize agitation). Agitation is not a common side effect of iloperidone, nor is there any indication that it may be more likely with fast titration.

B Incorrect (sedation). Although sedation can occur with iloperidone, the slow dose titration recommended for this medication is not associated with risk of sedation.

C Correct. Iloperidone has a very slow titration schedule in order to avoid orthostatic hypotension, which is theoretically due to its potent alpha 1 antagonism.

D Incorrect (prevent gastrointestinal upset). Gastrointestinal upset is not a particularly common side effect of iloperidone, and is not a factor in the slow titration schedule.

References

Schatzberg AF, Nemeroff CB. *Textbook of psychopharmacology*, fourth edition. Washington, DC: American Psychiatric Publishing, Inc.; 2009. (Chapters 28–33)

Stahl SM. *Essential psychopharmacology, the prescriber's guide*, fifth edition. New York, NY: Cambridge University Press; 2014.

Stahl SM. *Stahl's essential psychopharmacology*, fourth edition. New York, NY: Cambridge University Press; 2013. (Chapter 5)

Stahl SM, Mignon L. *Stahl's illustrated antipsychotics*, second edition. Carlsbad, CA: NEI Press; 2009. (Chapter 4)

QUESTION TEN

A patient who has been taking an atypical antipsychotic for 6 months has experienced a 22-pound weight gain since baseline. Which of the following pharmacologic properties most likely underlies this patient's metabolic changes?

A. Dopamine 2 antagonism

B. Serotonin 2A antagonism

C. Serotonin 2C antagonism

D. Alpha 1 adrenergic antagonism

Answer to Question Ten

The correct answer is C.

Choice	Peer answers
A. Dopamine 2 antagonism	0%
B. Serotonin 2A antagonism	8%
C. Serotonin 2C antagonism	83%
D. Alpha 1 adrenergic antagonism	8%

A Incorrect. Antagonism of dopamine 2 receptors is associated with both therapeutic and side effects, but is not linked to weight gain.

B Incorrect. Similarly, antagonism of serotonin 2A receptors has not been linked to risk for weight gain.

C Correct. Antagonism of serotonin 2C receptors is associated with increased risk for weight gain, perhaps in part due to stimulation of appetite regulated by the hypothalamus, and especially in combination with histamine 1 antagonism.

D Incorrect. Antagonism of alpha 1 adrenergic receptors is associated with side effects, but is not linked to weight gain.

References

Schatzberg AF, Nemeroff CB. *Textbook of psychopharmacology*, fourth edition. Washington, DC: American Psychiatric Publishing, Inc.; 2009. (Chapter 34)

Stahl SM. *Essential psychopharmacology, the prescriber's guide*, fifth edition. New York, NY: Cambridge University Press; 2014.

Stahl SM. *Stahl's essential psychopharmacology*, fourth edition. New York, NY: Cambridge University Press; 2013. (Chapter 5)

Stahl SM, Mignon L. *Stahl's illustrated antipsychotics*, second edition. Carlsbad, CA: NEI Press; 2009. (Chapter 3)

QUESTION ELEVEN

A 38-year-old woman was diagnosed with schizophrenia approximately 2 years ago and after multiple trials of different medications she has been maintained on haloperidol for the last several months with good response. Two weeks ago she began exhibiting mild motor symptoms of parkinsonism. Which of the following would be the most appropriate adjunct medication for this patient?

A. Cholinesterase inhibitor

B. Muscarinic 1 antagonist

C. Alpha 1 adrenergic agonist

D. Histamine 1 antagonist

Answer to Question Eleven

The correct answer is B.

Choice	Peer answers
A. Cholinesterase inhibitor	19%
B. Muscarinic 1 antagonist	63%
C. Alpha 1 adrenergic agonist	2%
D. Histamine 1 antagonist	16%

Extrapyramidal side effects (EPS) are associated with a relative deficiency of dopamine and an excess of acetylcholine in the nigrostriatal pathway. Increasing availability of dopamine and/or decreasing acetylcholine would therefore be expected to relieve EPS.

A Incorrect. A cholinesterase inhibitor would reduce metabolism of acetylcholine and cause a further increase, rather than decrease, in this neurotransmitter.

B Correct. On the other hand, antagonism of the muscarinic 1 receptor for acetylcholine would prevent it from binding there and thus reduce its effects, potentially relieving EPS.

C Incorrect. Haloperidol is an antagonist at the alpha 1 adrenergic receptor and an agonist would therefore reverse its effects; however, the adrenergic system is more often associated with a different form of EPS, akathisia, and thus actions here would not relieve the present symptoms (beta blockers can be used to treat akathisia).

D Incorrect. Similarly, the histamine system is not associated with development of or relief from EPS. Some antihistamines are muscarinic 1 antagonists but their H1 antagonist properties do not regulate EPS.

References

Schatzberg AF, Nemeroff CB. *Textbook of psychopharmacology*, fourth edition. Washington, DC: American Psychiatric Publishing, Inc.; 2009. (Chapter 34)

Stahl SM. *Essential psychopharmacology, the prescriber's guide*, fifth edition. New York, NY: Cambridge University Press; 2014.

Stahl SM. *Stahl's essential psychopharmacology*, fourth edition. New York, NY: Cambridge University Press; 2013. (Chapter 5)

Stahl SM, Mignon L. *Stahl's illustrated antipsychotics*, second edition. Carlsbad, CA: NEI Press; 2009. (Chapter 3)

QUESTION TWELVE

A 38-year-old man was diagnosed with schizophrenia 14 years ago, and over the course of his illness has taken several different antipsychotics, all with partial response and no severe side effects. He now presents with acute exacerbation of hallucinations and delusions. He recently had bowel resection due to a gastrointestinal disorder, and blood levels reveal that he is not absorbing his medications well. One option for this patient would be to prescribe heroic oral doses of his antipsychotic. Aside from this approach, which of the following antipsychotics have formulations that may be good long-term options for bypassing his problem with absorption?

A. Asenapine, paliperidone, risperidone

B. Paliperidone, risperidone, quetiapine

C. Risperidone, quetiapine, ziprasidone

D. Quetiapine, ziprasidone, asenapine

Answer to Question Twelve

The correct answer is A.

Choice	Peer answers
A. Asenapine, paliperidone, risperidone	79%
B. Paliperidone, risperidone, quetiapine	9%
C. Risperidone, quetiapine, ziprasidone	9%
D. Quetiapine, ziprasidone, asenapine	3%

A Correct (asenapine, paliperidone, risperidone). For patients with difficulty absorbing medications, the best options in order to reach therapeutic blood levels would be to prescribe heroic oral doses or to use parenteral, sublingual, or suppository administration. Asenapine has a sublingual formulation, while paliperidone is available in a 4-week and a 3-month formulation and risperidone is available as an intramuscular depot administered every 2 weeks. A 4-week olanzapine depot is also available. Additional antipsychotics with depot formulations include flupenthixol, fluphenazine, haloperidol, pipothiazine, and zuclopenthixol. Clozapine, olanzapine, and risperidone have orally disintegrating tablets; however, these medications are not absorbed sublingually and must be swallowed in order to undergo absorption in the gut. Chlorpromazine has a suppository formulation, and other antipsychotics may also be able to be administered as suppositories. Aripiprazole has two long-acting injectable formulations: one that is administered every 4 weeks and another that can be administered every 4 or 6 weeks. Iloperidone is in early trials for a 4-week depot.

B Incorrect (paliperidone, risperidone, quetiapine). Paliperidone and risperidone are both viable options, but quetiapine is only available as an oral tablet.

C Incorrect (risperidone, quetiapine, ziprasidone). Risperidone is a viable option. However, quetiapine is only available as an oral tablet. Ziprasidone is available in an intramuscular formulation, which would bypass absorption issues, but it is for acute agitation and is not to be administered long-term.

D Incorrect (quetiapine, ziprasidone, asenapine). Asenapine is a viable option, but neither quetiapine nor ziprasidone would be (see above for explanation).

References

Schatzberg AF, Nemeroff CB. *Textbook of psychopharmacology*, fourth edition. Washington, DC: American Psychiatric Publishing, Inc.; 2009. (Chapter 55)

Stahl SM. *Case studies: Stahl's essential psychopharmacology*. New York, NY: Cambridge University Press; 2011.

Stahl SM. *Essential psychopharmacology, the prescriber's guide*, fifth edition. New York, NY: Cambridge University Press; 2014.

Stahl SM. *Stahl's essential psychopharmacology*, fourth edition. New York, NY: Cambridge University Press; 2013. (Chapter 5)

Stahl SM, Mignon L. *Stahl's illustrated antipsychotics*, second edition. Carlsbad, CA: NEI Press; 2009. (Chapter 5)

Psychosis and schizophrenia and antipsychotics

QUESTION THIRTEEN

A 28-year-old man was recently diagnosed with schizophrenia. He has a body mass index of 30, fasting triglycerides of 220 mg/dL, and fasting glucose of 114 mg/dL. Which of the following is least likely to worsen his metabolic profile?

A. Olanzapine

B. Quetiapine

C. Risperidone

D. Ziprasidone

Answer to Question Thirteen

The correct answer is D.

Choice	Peer answers
A. Olanzapine	9%
B. Quetiapine	10%
C. Risperidone	3%
D. Ziprasidone	78%

A Incorrect. Olanzapine is one of the antipsychotics most associated with weight gain and metabolic risk and would not be a first-line option for patients who have a primary concern about metabolic issues.

B Incorrect. Quetiapine can lead to weight gain and increased triglyceride levels and may be a second-line option if a primary concern is metabolic issues.

C Incorrect. Risperidone can lead to weight gain and increased triglyceride levels and may be a second-line option if a primary concern is metabolic issues.

D Correct. Ziprasidone in general seems to be weight neutral and has been shown to lower triglyceride levels. It is therefore a recommended choice for individuals for whom metabolic issues are a primary concern.

References

Schatzberg AF, Nemeroff CB. *Textbook of psychopharmacology*, fourth edition. Washington, DC: American Psychiatric Publishing, Inc.; 2009. (Chapter 55)

Stahl SM. *Case studies: Stahl's essential psychopharmacology*. New York, NY: Cambridge University Press; 2011.

Stahl SM. *Essential psychopharmacology, the prescriber's guide*, fifth edition. New York, NY: Cambridge University Press; 2014.

Stahl SM. *Stahl's essential psychopharmacology*, fourth edition. New York, NY: Cambridge University Press; 2013. (Chapter 5)

Stahl SM, Mignon L. *Stahl's illustrated antipsychotics*, second edition. Carlsbad, CA: NEI Press; 2009. (Chapter 5)

QUESTION FOURTEEN

A 27-year-old male who has been treated with risperidone for the last 8 weeks is now having his medication changed to quetiapine. What is the recommended switching method in this situation, assuming the need to do this expeditiously, but not urgently, as an outpatient?

A. Maintain therapeutic dose of risperidone while uptitrating quetiapine to effective dose, then discontinue risperidone

B. Down-titrate risperidone over several weeks while uptitrating quetiapine over the same time period

C. Down-titrate risperidone over at least 1 week while uptitrating quetiapine over at least 2 weeks

D. Down-titrate risperidone over at least 2 weeks while uptitrating quetiapine over 1 week

Answer to Question Fourteen

The correct answer is C.

Choice	Peer answers
A. Maintain therapeutic dose of risperidone while uptitrating quetiapine to effective dose, then discontinue risperidone	11%
B. Down-titrate risperidone over several weeks while uptitrating quetiapine over the same time period	19%
C. Down-titrate risperidone over at least 1 week while uptitrating quetiapine over at least 2 weeks	49%
D. Down-titrate risperidone over at least 2 weeks while uptitrating quetiapine over 1 week	21%

A Incorrect. Maintain therapeutic dose of risperidone while uptitrating quetiapine to an effective dose, then discontinue risperidone: It is not generally recommended to maintain full therapeutic dose of one antipsychotic while uptitrating another as this can cause increased risk of side effects.

B Incorrect. Down-titrate risperidone over several weeks while uptitrating quetiapine over the same time period: In general cross-titration with risperidone and quetiapine would not have to be this slow.

C Correct. Down-titrate risperidone over at least 1 week while uptitrating quetiapine over at least 2 weeks: Tolerability may be best if quetiapine can be titrated up over the course of 2 weeks, while keeping the estimated D2 receptor occupancy constant as the risperidone is stopped.

D Incorrect. Down-titrate risperidone over at least 2 weeks while uptitrating quetiapine over 1 week: Risperidone can be down-titrated faster than this. In addition, tolerability may be best if uptitration of quetiapine is slower.

References

Schatzberg AF, Nemeroff CB. *Textbook of psychopharmacology*, fourth edition. Washington, DC: American Psychiatric Publishing, Inc.; 2009. (Chapter 55)

Stahl SM. *Case studies: Stahl's essential psychopharmacology*. New York, NY: Cambridge University Press; 2011.

Stahl SM. *Essential psychopharmacology, the prescriber's guide*, fifth edition. New York, NY: Cambridge University Press; 2014.

Stahl SM. *Stahl's essential psychopharmacology*, fourth edition. New York, NY: Cambridge University Press; 2013. (Chapter 5)

Stahl SM, Mignon L. *Stahl's illustrated antipsychotics*, second edition. Carlsbad, CA: NEI Press; 2009. (Chapter 5)

QUESTION FIFTEEN

A 16-year-old female is brought to the hospital by her mother because she is complaining that her neighbors spy on her and submit their observations to the government. After evaluation, she is diagnosed with schizophrenia and prescribed risperidone. Which of the following is the appropriate target therapeutic dose for this patient?

A. 0.5 mg/day

B. 3 mg/day

C. 6 mg/day

D. 12 mg/day

Answer to Question Fifteen

The correct answer is B.

Choice	Peer answers
A. 0.5 mg/day	9%
B. 3 mg/day	65%
C. 6 mg/day	26%
D. 12 mg/day	0%

A Incorrect. 0.5 mg/day: Although this is the recommended starting dose for adolescents with schizophrenia (ages 13 to 17), the recommended therapeutic dose is higher.

B Correct. 3 mg/day: This is the recommended therapeutic dose for adolescents (ages 13 to 17) with schizophrenia.

C Incorrect. 6 mg/day: This is within the recommended dose range for adults with schizophrenia; however, in studies of adolescents doses above 3 mg/day were associated with additional side effects and no additional efficacy.

D Incorrect. 12 mg/day: Doses above 6 mg/day have not been studied in adolescents with schizophrenia.

References

Schatzberg AF, Nemeroff CB. *Textbook of psychopharmacology*, fourth edition. Washington, DC: American Psychiatric Publishing, Inc.; 2009. (Chapters 62–65)

Stahl SM. *Essential psychopharmacology*, the prescriber's guide, fifth edition. New York, NY: Cambridge University Press; 2014.

Stahl SM. *Stahl's essential psychopharmacology*, fourth edition. New York, NY: Cambridge University Press; 2013. (Chapter 5)

QUESTION SIXTEEN

A 27-year-old male who has been treated with quetiapine for the last 8 weeks is now having his medication changed to aripiprazole. What is the recommended starting dose for aripiprazole?

A. Low dose

B. Middle dose

C. Full dose

Answer to Question Sixteen

The correct answer is B.

Choice	Peer answers
A. Low dose	28%
B. Middle dose	60%
C. Full dose	12%

B Correct. When switching from quetiapine (or asenapine or olanzapine) to aripiprazole, the "pine" should be tapered over 3 to 4 weeks to allow patients to readapt to the withdrawal of blocking cholinergic, histaminic, and alpha-1 receptors. This should help reduce the risk of agitation or rebound psychosis. In addition, a benzodiazepine or anticholinergic medication can be administered to help alleviate these effects if they occur. Aripiprazole can be initiated at a **middle** dose and titrated up over 1 to 2 weeks, so that it reaches full dose while the pine is still being tapered. This results in short-term polypharmacy; however, the pine should ultimately be discontinued completely.

A Incorrect (low dose).

C Incorrect (full dose).

References

Stahl SM. *Essential psychopharmacology, the prescriber's guide*, fifth edition. New York, NY: Cambridge University Press; 2014.

Stahl SM. *Stahl's essential psychopharmacology*, fourth edition. New York, NY: Cambridge University Press; 2013. (Chapter 5)

Psychosis and schizophrenia and antipsychotics

QUESTION SEVENTEEN

A 44-year-old woman with schizophrenia and a history of depression has developed tardive dyskinesia after taking haloperidol 15 mg/day for 2 years. Which of the following would be the most appropriate pharmacologic option to manage her tardive dyskinesia?

A. Amantadine

B. Benztropine

C. Clonazepam

D. Reserpine

Answer to Question Seventeen

The correct answer is C.

Choice	Peer answers
A. Amantadine	51%
B. Benztropine	39%
C. Clonazepam	2%
D. Reserpine	9%

Tardive dyskinesia will reverse in approximately one-third of patients over a 6-month period after the offending medication is discontinued. For patients who do not experience reversal of their tardive dyskinesia, there are augmentation options to treat it.

A Incorrect. Amantadine is a dopamine agonist with preliminary evidence of efficacy in treating tardive dyskinesia. Although it is not recommended first-line (clonazepam has the best evidence of efficacy), it would be a reasonable second-line choice for this patient.

B Incorrect. Benztropine is a central anticholinergic medication; such agents can improve drug-induced parkinsonism but exacerbate or unmask tardive dyskinesia. This effect may be reversible if the anticholinergic medication is discontinued.

C Correct. According to a recent review by the American Academy of Neurology, the treatments with the best evidence of efficacy for tardive dyskinesia are clonazepam and ginkgo biloba.

D Incorrect. Reserpine is a dopamine-depleting agent and has historically been considered a first-line treatment for tardive dyskinesia. However, it is contraindicated in patients with a history of depression and thus would not be appropriate for this patient.

References

Aia PG, Reveulta GJ, Cloud LJ, Factor SA. Tardive dyskinesia. *Curr Treat Options Neurol* 2011;**13**(3):231–41.

Bhidayasiri R, Fahn S, Weiner WJ, et al. Evidence-based guideline: treatment of tardive syndromes: report of the Guideline Development Subcommittee of the American Academy of Neurology. *Neurology* 2013;**81**(5):463–9.

Psychosis and schizophrenia and antipsychotics

QUESTION EIGHTEEN

Carol is a 47-year-old patient with schizophrenia. She was taking a conventional antipsychotic but decided to stop taking it when she developed parkinsonian symptoms. Secondary to stopping her conventional antipsychotic, Carol's auditory hallucinations and paranoia returned, and she was rehospitalized. You recommend that she be started on an atypical antipsychotic. Which of the following has the lowest risk of extrapyramidal symptoms associated with it?

A. Asenapine

B. Iloperidone

C. Olanzapine

D. Paliperidone

Answer to Question Eighteen

The correct answer is B.

Choice	Peer answers
A. Asenapine	16%
B. Iloperidone	43%
C. Olanzapine	36%
D. Paliperidone	5%

As a class, atypical antipsychotics tend to have a decreased risk of movement disorders relative to conventional antipsychotics; however, the risk differs with each individual agent.

A Incorrect (asenapine).

B Correct. Of the agents listed here, iloperidone has a relatively lower risk of EPS. Other agents with a relatively lower risk of EPS include clozapine and quetiapine.

C Incorrect (olanzapine).

D Incorrect (paliperidone).

References

Roth BL. Ki determinations, receptor binding profiles, agonist and/or antagonist functional data, HERG data, MDR1 data, etc. as appropriate were generously provided by the National Institute of Mental Health's Psychoactive Drug Screening Program, Contract # HHSN-271–2008-00025-C (NIMH PDSP). The NIMH PDSP is directed by Bryan L. Roth MD, PhD at the University of North Carolina at Chapel Hill and Project Officer Jamie Driscol at NIMH, Bethesda MD, USA. For experimental details please refer to the PDSP website http://pdsp.med.unc.edu.

Santana N, Mengod G, Artigas F. Expression of alpha 1-adrenergic receptors in rat prefrontal cortex: cellular co-localization with 5-HT2A receptors. *Int J Neuropsychopharmacol* 2013;**16**(5):1139–51.

Stahl SM. *Stahl's essential psychopharmacology*, fourth edition. New York, NY: Cambridge University Press; 2013.

QUESTION NINETEEN

A 34-year-old man who has been taking a conventional anti-psychotic for 6 years has begun demonstrating extrapyramidal side effects (EPS), and his clinician elects to switch him to an atypical antipsychotic with serotonin 2A antagonism. The majority of atypical antipsychotics:

A. Have higher affinity for dopamine 2 receptors than for serotonin 2A receptors

B. Have higher affinity for serotonin 2A receptors than for dopamine 2 receptors

Answer to Question Nineteen

The correct answer is B.

Choice	Peer answers
A. Have higher affinity for dopamine 2 receptors than for serotonin 2A receptors	25%
B. Have higher affinity for serotonin 2A receptors than for dopamine 2 receptors	75%

B Correct. Theoretically, low EPS has been linked to high affinity for blocking serotonin 2A receptors. Because nearly all atypical antipsychotics have actions at serotonin 2A receptors, it may be beneficial to understand how stimulating or blocking these receptors can regulate dopamine release.

Serotonin neurons originate in the raphe nucleus of the brainstem and project throughout the brain, including to the cortex. They synapse there with glutamatergic pyramidal neurons, which project to the substantia nigra in the brainstem. The substantia nigra is the origin of dopaminergic neurons that project to the striatum. All serotonin 2A receptors are postsynaptic. When they are located on cortical pyramidal neurons, they are excitatory. Thus, when serotonin is released in the cortex and binds to serotonin 2A receptors on glutamatergic pyramidal neurons, this stimulates them to release glutamate in the brainstem, which in turn stimulates GABA release. GABA binds to dopaminergic neurons projecting from the substantia nigra to the striatum, inhibiting dopamine release and possibly leading to EPS and akathisia.

Nearly all atypical antipsychotics have an affinity for blocking serotonin 2A receptors that is equal to or greater than their affinity for blocking dopamine 2 receptors. The "pines" – clozapine, olanzapine, quetiapine, and asenapine – all bind much more potently to the serotonin 2A receptor than they do to the dopamine 2 receptor. The "dones" – risperidone, paliperidone, ziprasidone, iloperidone, and lurasidone – also bind more potently to the serotonin 2A receptor than to the dopamine 2 receptor, or show similar potency at both receptors. Aripiprazole binds more potently to the dopamine 2 receptor than to the serotonin 2A receptor; however, it is also a partial agonist at dopamine 2 receptors, which may contribute to its lower propensity to induce EPS.

A Incorrect (have higher affinity for serotonin 2A receptors than for dopamine 2 receptors).

Psychosis and schizophrenia and antipsychotics

References

Roth BL. Ki determinations, receptor binding profiles, agonist and/or antagonist functional data, HERG data, MDR1 data, etc. as appropriate were generously provided by the National Institute of Mental Health's Psychoactive Drug Screening Program, Contract # HHSN-271–2008–00025-C (NIMH PDSP). The NIMH PDSP is directed by Bryan L. Roth MD, PhD at the University of North Carolina at Chapel Hill and Project Officer Jamie Driscol at NIMH, Bethesda MD, USA. For experimental details please refer to the PDSP website http://pdsp.med.unc.edu.

Stahl SM. *Stahl's essential psychopharmacology*, fourth edition. New York, NY: Cambridge University Press; 2013.

QUESTION TWENTY

Reggie is a 30-year-old male patient with schizophrenia. He is currently taking iloperidone 24 mg/day as well as aripiprazole 15 mg/day but continues to experience visual hallucinations. To improve this patient's psychosis, it is likely necessary to further increase the blockade of dopamine D2 receptors. Which treatment strategy is likely the best course of action?

A. Increase iloperidone dose while keeping aripiprazole dose the same

B. Increase iloperidone and aripiprazole doses

C. Increase aripiprazole dose while keeping iloperidone dose the same

D. Maintain iloperidone dose and discontinue aripiprazole

Answer to Question Twenty

The correct answer is D.

Choice	Peer answers
A. Increase iloperidone dose while keeping aripiprazole dose the same	12%
B. Increase iloperidone and aripiprazole doses	0%
C. Increase aripiprazole dose while keeping iloperidone dose the same	37%
D. Maintain iloperidone dose and discontinue aripiprazole	51%

Aripiprazole is unique among antipsychotics because it is a dopamine D2 partial agonist as well as one of the most potent agents that bind to D2 receptors. Thus, when given concomitantly with a D2 antagonist, such as iloperidone, it can actually reduce the level of D2 blockade compared to D2 antagonist monotherapy, thus reducing the antipsychotic efficacy.

A Incorrect. Increasing the dose of iloperidone while maintaining the aripiprazole dose would not likely lead to a relevant increase in D2 blockade (and corresponding improvement of psychotic symptoms), since aripiprazole has higher affinity for the D2 receptor.

B Incorrect. Increasing doses of both iloperidone and aripiprazole would not likely lead to improvement of psychotic symptoms, since aripiprazole would continue to compete with iloperidone at the D2 receptor.

C Incorrect. Increasing the dose of aripiprazole may actually decrease D2 blockade rather than increase it, since aripiprazole has higher affinity for the D2 receptor than iloperidone.

D Correct. Because aripiprazole may be reducing the level of D2 blockade relative to iloperidone monotherapy, the best strategy for increasing D2 blockade (and correspondingly improving psychotic symptoms) may be to use monotherapy.

References
Stahl SM. *Stahl's essential psychopharmacology*, fourth edition. New York, NY: Cambridge University Press; 2013.

Chapter peer comparison

For the Psychosis and schizophrenia and antipsychotics section, the correct answer was selected 63% of the time.

3   UNIPOLAR DEPRESSION AND ANTIDEPRESSANTS

QUESTION ONE

A 26-year-old woman began treatment for a major depressive episode 8 months ago. Two months into her treatment she began to experience noticeable symptom improvement, and for the last 5 months she has been nearly symptom free. According to the general consensus, her current state could be classified as a:

A. Response

B. Remission

C. Recovery

D. Relapse

E. Recurrence

Answer to Question One

The correct answer is B.

Choice	Peer answers
A. Response	16%
B. Remission	81%
C. Recovery	3%
D. Relapse	0%
E. Recurrence	0%

A Incorrect. A response is characterized as at least a 50% improvement of symptoms, whereas this patient has experienced a near elimination of symptoms.

B Correct. When treatment of depression results in removal of essentially all symptoms, as with this patient, it is called remission for the first several months (e.g., up to 6 months).

C Incorrect. Recovery is described as being symptom-free for 6 months or more.

D Incorrect. When depression returns before there is a full remission of symptoms or within the first several months following remission of symptoms, it is called a relapse.

E Incorrect. When depression symptoms return after a patient has recovered, it is called a recurrence.

References

Schatzberg AF, Nemeroff CB. *Textbook of psychopharmacology*, fourth edition. Washington, DC: American Psychiatric Publishing, Inc.; 2009. (Chapter 53)

Stahl SM. *Stahl's essential psychopharmacology*, fourth edition. New York, NY: Cambridge University Press; 2013. (Chapter 7)

Zimmerman M, McGlinchey JB, Posternak MA, Friedman M, Attiullah N, Boerescu D. How should remission from depression be defined? The depressed patient's perspective. *Am J Psychiatry* 2006;**163**:148–50.

QUESTION TWO

A 38-year-old patient with depression presents with depressed mood, anhedonia, and loss of energy. These symptoms can be conceptualized as reflecting reduced positive affect; such a categorization is theoretically useful because it may direct treatment choice. Specifically, symptoms of reduced positive affect are hypothetically more likely to respond to agents that enhance:

A. Serotonin and possibly dopamine function

B. Dopamine and possibly norepinephrine function

C. Norepinephrine and possibly serotonin function

Answer to Question Two

The correct answer is B.

Choice	Peer answers
A. Serotonin and possibly dopamine function	2%
B. Dopamine and possibly norepinephrine function	61%
C. Norepinephrine and possibly serotonin function	17%

Mood-related symptoms of depression can be characterized by their affective expression – that is, whether they cause a reduction in positive affect (e.g., depressed mood, anhedonia) or an increase in negative affect (e.g., anxiety, irritability). This concept is based on the fact that there are diffuse anatomic connections of monoamines throughout the brain, with diffuse dopamine dysfunction in this system driving predominantly the reduction of positive affect, diffuse serotonin dysfunction driving predominantly the increase in negative affect, and norepinephrine dysfunction being involved in both.

A   Incorrect. Although dopaminergic dysfunction is thought to be related to decreased positive affect, serotonergic dysfunction is thought to be related to increased negative affect.

B   Correct. Because reduced positive affect is thought to be related to dopamine dysfunction and possibly norepinephrine dysfunction, enhancing one or both of these neurotransmitters would theoretically be most likely to improve these symptoms.

C   Incorrect. Although norepinephrine dysfunction is thought to be involved in reduced positive affect, serotonergic dysfunction is thought be related to increased negative affect.

References

Schatzberg AF, Nemeroff CB. *Textbook of psychopharmacology*, fourth edition. Washington, DC: American Psychiatric Publishing, Inc.; 2009. (Chapter 45)

Stahl SM. *Stahl's essential psychopharmacology*, fourth edition. New York, NY: Cambridge University Press; 2013. (Chapter 7)

QUESTION THREE

A 36-year-old man with major depressive disorder is having lab work done to assess his levels of inflammatory markers. Based on the current evidence regarding inflammation in depression, which of the following results would you most likely suspect for this patient?

A. Elevated levels of tumor necrosis factor-alpha (TNF-alpha)

B. Reduced levels of interleukin 6 (IL-6)

C. Both A and B

D. Neither A nor B

Answer to Question Three

The correct answer is A.

Choice	Peer answers
A. Elevated levels of tumor necrosis factor-alpha (TNF-alpha)	52%
B. Reduced levels of interleukin 6 (IL-6)	9%
C. Both A and B	28%
D. Neither A nor B	11%

A Correct. There is growing evidence that inflammation may play an important role in the pathophysiology of major depression. Clinical studies have shown that depressed patients have significantly higher concentrations of several inflammatory markers, including the pro-inflammatory cytokines TNF-alpha, interleukin 6, and interleukin 1. Patients with depression also have higher concentrations of C-reactive protein, which is synthesized by the liver in response to pro-inflammatory cytokines. Furthermore, both cytokines and cytokine inducers can cause symptoms of depression. For example, as many as 50% of patients receiving chronic therapy with the cytokine interferon develop symptoms consistent with idiopathic depression.

B, C, and D Incorrect.

References

Dowlati Y, Herrmann N, Swardfager JW, et al. A meta-analysis of cytokines in major depression. *Biol Psychiatry* 2010;**67**:446–57.

Haroon E, Raison CL, Miller AH. Psychoneuroimmunology meets neuropsychopharmacology: translational implications of the impact of inflammation on behavior. *Neuropsychopharmacology* 2012;**37**:137–62.

Howren MB, Lamkin DM, Suls J. Associations of depression with C-reactive protein, IL-1, and IL-6: a meta-analysis. *Psychosom Med* 2009;**71**:171–86.

Raison CL, Miller AH. Is depression an inflammatory disorder? *Curr Psychiatry Rep* 2011;**13**:467–75.

QUESTION FOUR

A 36-year-old man with major depressive disorder has lab work done to assess his levels of inflammatory markers. The results come back indicating elevated levels of tumor necrosis factor-alpha (TNF-alpha) and interleukin 6 (IL-6). Elevated cytokine levels may indirectly lead to:

A. Excessive glutamate and reduced serotonin

B. Excessive glutamate and excessive serotonin

C. Reduced glutamate and reduced serotonin

D. Reduced glutamate and excessive serotonin

Answer to Question Four

The correct answer is A.

Choice	Peer answers
A. Excessive glutamate and reduced serotonin	73%
B. Excessive glutamate and excessive serotonin	2%
C. Reduced glutamate and reduced serotonin	23%
D. Reduced glutamate and excessive serotonin	2%

A Correct. Cytokines can influence neurotransmitter levels, including both serotonin and glutamate. Normally, tryptophan is converted into 5-hydroxytryptophan, which is then converted into serotonin. However, tryptophan can also be broken down by the enzyme indoleamine 2,3 dioxygenase (IDO), resulting in kynurenine production. Kynurenine is then converted into quinolinic acid, which is an NMDA agonist and thus leads to increased glutamate. Cytokines, such as interleukin 6, tumor necrosis factor-alpha, and interferon gamma, can activate IDO. Thus, when levels of these cytokines are elevated, the increased activation of IDO may lead to a depletion of tryptophan, with a corresponding *decrease in serotonin synthesis*. In addition, the increased activation of IDO would lead to increased synthesis of quinolinic acid. This could potentially result in *excessive glutamate* activity and oxidative stress. In fact, excessive glutamate activity is hypothesized to be an underlying cause of depression.

B, C, and D Incorrect.

References

Dowlati Y, Herrmann N, Swardfager JW, et al. A meta-analysis of cytokines in major depression. *Biol Psychiatry* 2010;**67**:446–57.

Haroon E, Raison CL, Miller AH. Psychoneuroimmunology meets neuropsychopharmacology: translational implications of the impact of inflammation on behavior. *Neuropsychopharmacology* 2012;**37**:137–62.

Howren MB, Lamkin DM, Suls J. Associations of depression with C-reactive protein, IL-1, and IL-6: a meta-analysis. *Psychosom Med* 2009;**71**:171–86.

Raison CL, Miller AH. Is depression an inflammatory disorder? *Curr Psychiatry Rep* 2011;**13**:467–75.

QUESTION FIVE

A 44-year-old man taking paroxetine for depression reports experiencing sexual dysfunction. He opts to discontinue pharmacotherapy, at which time he experiences akathisia and dizziness. Which of the following properties may be responsible for the side effects and withdrawal effects that he has experienced?

A. Inhibition of CYP450 3A4

B. Inhibition of nitric oxide synthetase (NOS)

C. Anticholinergic actions

D. A and B

E. B and C

Answer to Question Five

The correct answer is E.

Choice	Peer answers
A. Inhibition of CYP450 3A4	9%
B. Inhibition of nitric oxide synthetase (NOS)	12%
C. Anticholinergic actions	24%
D. A and B	9%
E. B and C	45%

A and D Incorrect. Inhibition of CYP450 3A4 is not part of paroxetine's pharmacokinetic profile. However, since paroxetine is a substrate and an inhibitor of 2D6, this can lead to a rapid decline in plasma drug levels when paroxetine is discontinued, which can contribute to withdrawal symptoms.

B and C Correct. Inhibition of NOS may contribute to the sexual dysfunction this patient has experienced. Anticholinergic actions of paroxetine may be responsible for the patient's experience of akathisia and dizziness due to anticholinergic rebound when paroxetine is discontinued.

E Correct, as B and C are both correct answers.

References

Schatzberg AF, Nemeroff CB. *Textbook of psychopharmacology*, fourth edition. Washington, DC: American Psychiatric Publishing, Inc.; 2009. (Chapters 13–17, 19, 21–23)

Stahl SM. *Stahl's essential psychopharmacology*, fourth edition. New York, NY: Cambridge University Press; 2013. (Chapter 7)

Stahl SM. *Stahl's essential psychopharmacology*, the prescriber's guide, fifth edition. New York, NY: Cambridge University Press; 2014.

QUESTION SIX

Denise is a 56-year-old perimenopausal patient with a history of depression. Her depressed mood seems to be responding to her current treatment with the selective serotonin reuptake inhibitor (SSRI) fluoxetine (40 mg/day); however, she is troubled by hot flashes and night sweats, and she reports some residual depressed mood. Which treatment strategy is likely to optimize this patient's chance for remission?

A. Maintain current fluoxetine dose

B. Decrease fluoxetine dose

C. Switch to a different selective serotonin reuptake inhibitor (SSRI)

D. Switch to a serotonin and norepinephrine reuptake inhibitor (SNRI)

Answer to Question Six

The correct answer is D.

Choice	Peer answers
A. Maintain current fluoxetine dose	7%
B. Decrease fluoxetine dose	2%
C. Switch to a different selective serotonin reuptake inhibitor (SSRI)	11%
D. Switch to a serotonin and norepinephrine reuptake inhibitor (SNRI)	79%

D Correct. Vasomotor symptoms, including hot flashes and night sweats, are associated with estrogen fluctuations, such as those that occur during the perimenopausal period of the female lifespan. Estrogen fluctuations lead to dysregulation of the serotonergic and noradrenergic systems that are thought to mediate both vasomotor symptoms and depression. Vasomotor symptoms may signal vulnerability to the onset or recurrence of a major depressive episode; this is not surprising because the presence of vasomotor symptoms indicates that estrogen is in flux even if depressive symptoms are responding to antidepressant treatment. Although SSRIs may have some efficacy in the treatment of both depression and vasomotor symptoms, SNRIs have been shown to be more effective and are the treatment of choice for patients with these symptoms.

A Incorrect. The ultimate goal of depression treatment should be the amelioration of all symptoms rather than improvement in depressive symptoms alone. Residual symptoms are often predictive of poor long-term outcomes, including increased disability, more frequent relapses, relationship and work difficulties, and suicide. Although this patient is responding to her current treatment with fluoxetine, she is experiencing residual depressed mood and vasomotor symptoms. The presence of vasomotor symptoms indicates that this patient's estrogen levels are in flux, putting her at risk for depressive relapse. In order to prevent relapse and achieve remission, a change in treatment strategy is warranted.

B Incorrect. This patient is having at least partial response to her current dose of fluoxetine. Decreasing the dose is likely to diminish the therapeutic effects of fluoxetine and not improve her vasomotor symptoms.

C Incorrect. Vasomotor symptoms are thought to be due to dysfunction in both serotonin and norepinephrine neurotransmission, specifically in the hypothalamus. Although SSRIs may have some

Unipolar depression and antidepressants

efficacy in the treatment of both depression and vasomotor symptoms, SNRIs have been shown to be more effective and are the treatment of choice for patients with these symptoms.

References

Schatzberg AF, Nemeroff CB. *Textbook of psychopharmacology*, fourth edition. Washington, DC: American Psychiatric Publishing, Inc.; 2009. (Chapters 62–65)

Stahl SM. Vasomotor symptoms and depression in women, part 1: role of vasomotor symptoms in signaling the onset or relapse of a major depressive episode. *J Clin Psychiatry* 2009;**70**(1):11–12.

Stahl SM. Vasomotor symptoms and depression in women, part 2: treatments that cause remission and prevent relapses of major depressive episodes overlap with treatments for vasomotor symptoms. *J Clin Psychiatry* 2009;**70**(3):310–11.

Unipolar depression and antidepressants

QUESTION SEVEN

Margaret is a 42-year-old patient with untreated depression. She is reluctant to begin antidepressant treatment due to concerns about treatment-induced weight gain. Which of the following anti-depressant treatments is associated with the greatest risk of weight gain?

A. Escitalopram

B. Fluoxetine

C. Mirtazapine

D. Vilazodone

Answer to Question Seven

The correct answer is C.

Choice	Peer answers
A. Escitalopram	1%
B. Fluoxetine	5%
C. Mirtazapine	94%
D. Vilazodone	0%

A Incorrect. Although weight gain may occur, it is not commonly reported with escitalopram, and a meta-analysis suggests that the risk of both short- and long-term weight gain with escitalopram is low.

B Incorrect. Although weight gain may occur, it is not commonly reported with fluoxetine and a meta-analysis did not find significant increase in weight over the short- or long-term. Some patients actually experience short-term weight loss with fluoxetine.

C Correct. Meta-analysis has shown that mirtazapine, an alpha 2 antagonist, may cause both short- and long-term weight gain. This is consistent with its secondary pharmacologic properties: mirtazapine is an antagonist at both serotonin 2C and histamine 1 receptors, the combination of which has been proposed to cause weight gain. However, it should be noted that average weight gain with any antidepressant is small, and rather than a widespread effect it may instead be that a small number of individuals experience significant weight gain due to their genetic predispositions and other factors.

D Incorrect. Although weight gain may occur, studies with vilazodone have suggested a lower risk for weight gain compared to many other antidepressants that block serotonin reuptake; however, head-to-head studies have not been conducted.

References
Serretti A, Mandelli L. Antidepressants and body weight: a comprehensive review and meta-analysis. *J Clin Psychiatry* 2010;**71**(10):1259–72.

Stahl SM. *Essential psychopharmacology, the prescriber's guide*, fifth edition. New York, NY: Cambridge University Press; 2014.

Unipolar depression and antidepressants

QUESTION EIGHT

A 52-year-old man presents to the emergency room with symptoms of hypertensive crisis after an evening dining out with friends. He is currently taking a monoamine oxidase inhibitor (MAOI). Which of the following foods must be avoided by patients taking MAOIs?

A. Fresh fish

B. Aged cheese

C. Bottled beer

D. All of these must be avoided

E. None of these must be avoided

Answer to Question Eight

The correct answer is B.

Choice	Peer answers
A. Fresh fish	0%
B. Aged cheese	83%
C. Bottled beer	0%
D. All of these must be avoided	16%
E. None of these must be avoided	1%

Tyramine content in food can instigate a hypertensive crisis in patients taking MAOIs. Meals considered to contain a high level of tyramine content generally include 40 mg of tyramine.

Foods to AVOID*	Foods ALLOWED
Dried, aged, smoked, fermented, spoiled, or improperly stored meat, poultry, and fish	Fresh or processed meat, poultry, and fish
Broad bean pods	All other vegetables
Aged cheeses	Processed cheese slices, cottage cheese, ricotta cheese, cream cheese, yogurt
Tap and unpasteurized beer	Bottled or canned beer and alcohol
Marmite	Brewer's and baker's yeast
Soy products/tofu	Peanuts
Banana peel	Bananas, avocados, raspberries
Sauerkraut, kimchee	
Tyramine-containing nutritional supplements	

* Not necessary for 6-mg transdermal or low-dose oral selegiline.

A   Incorrect. Fresh fish does not have a high tyramine content and can therefore be safely consumed when one is taking an MAOI.

B   Correct. Aged cheeses in general have a high tyramine content and must be avoided when a patient is taking an MAOI.

C   Incorrect. Bottled beer does not have a high tyramine content and can therefore be safely consumed when one is taking an MAOI.

D and E   Incorrect.

References

Shulman KI, Walker SE, MacKenzie S, Knowles S. Dietary restriction, tyramine, and the use of monoamine oxidase inhibitors. *J Clin Psychopharmacol* 1989;**9**(6):397–402.

Shulman KI, Walker SE. Refining the MAOI diet: tyramine content of pizzas and soy products. *J Clin Psychiatry* 1999;**60**(3):191–3.

Shulman KI, Walker SE. A reevaluation of dietary restrictions for irreversible monoamine oxidase inhibitors. *Psychiatr Ann* 2001;**31**(6):378–84.

QUESTION NINE

A 48-year-old woman with a history of treatment-resistant depression is currently taking duloxetine 60 mg/day with partial response as well as trazodone 50 mg/day for insomnia. She states that she feels empty and useless, and she admits to having thoughts of death. She states that she does not have plans to kill herself because it would harm her family and pets. Her clinician decides to try tranylcypromine, a monoamine oxidase inhibitor (MAOI) and one of the few agents that she has not yet tried. Which of the patient's current medications would you discontinue BEFORE initiating tranylcypromine?

A. Duloxetine

B. Trazodone

C. Both duloxetine and trazodone

D. Neither duloxetine nor trazodone

Answer to Question Nine

The correct answer is A.

Choice	Peer answers
A. Duloxetine	42%
B. Trazodone	2%
C. Both duloxetine and trazodone	55%
D. Neither duloxetine nor trazodone	1%

A Correct. Duloxetine is a serotonin norepinephrine reuptake inhibitor. Inhibition of the serotonin transporter leads to increased synaptic availability of serotonin. Similarly, inhibition of MAO leads to increased serotonin levels. In combination, these two mechanisms can cause excessive stimulation of postsynaptic serotonin receptors, which has the potential to cause a fatal "serotonin syndrome" or "serotonin toxicity." Because of the risk of serotonin toxicity, complete washout of duloxetine is necessary before starting an MAOI. Duloxetine must be down-titrated as tolerated, after which one must wait 5 half-lives of duloxetine (at least 3–4 days) before initiating the MAOI.

B Incorrect. Although trazodone does have serotonin reuptake inhibition at antidepressant doses (150 mg or higher), this property is not clinically relevant at the low doses used for insomnia. In fact, because there is a required gap in antidepressant treatment when switching to or from an MAO inhibitor, low-dose trazodone can be useful as a bridging agent when switching.

C and D Incorrect.

References

Dvir Y, Smallwood P. Serotonin syndrome: a complex but easily avoidable condition. *Gen Hosp Psychiatry* 2008;**30**(3):284–7.

Stahl SM. *Stahl's essential psychopharmacology*, fourth edition. New York, NY: Cambridge University Press; 2013. (Chapter 7)

Stahl SM. *Essential psychopharmacology, the prescriber's guide*, fifth edition. New York, NY: Cambridge University Press; 2014.

Wimbiscus M, Kostenkjo O, Malone D. MAO inhibitors: risks, benefits, and lore. *Cleveland Clinic J Med* 2010;**77**(12):859–82.

QUESTION TEN

A 56-year-old male patient with major depression is brought to the ER with cardiac arrhythmia and possible cardiac arrest. While at the hospital, he suffers a seizure. His wife states that he may have ingested an increased dose of his medication. Which of the following is most likely responsible for this apparent overdose reaction?

A. Clomipramine

B. Atomoxetine

C. Fluvoxamine

D. Venlafaxine

Answer to Question Ten

The correct answer is A.

Choice	Peer answers
A. Clomipramine	76%
B. Atomoxetine	7%
C. Fluvoxamine	5%
D. Venlafaxine	12%

A Correct. Clomipramine, a tricyclic antidepressant (TCA), may be most likely to cause these effects in overdose. TCAs block voltage-sensitive sodium channels (VSSCs) in both the brain and the heart. This action is weak at therapeutic doses, but in overdose may lead to coma, seizures, and cardiac arrhythmia, and may even prove fatal.

B Incorrect. Atomoxetine, a norepinephrine reuptake inhibitor, does not block VSSCs and is not noted to have severe cardiac impairments upon overdose; rather, sedation, agitation, hyperactivity, abnormal behavior, and GI symptoms are most commonly reported.

C Incorrect. Fluvoxamine, a selective serotonin reuptake inhibitor (SSRI), also does not block VSSCs and does not generally cause severe cardiac impairment in overdose.

D Incorrect. Venlafaxine is a serotonin-norepinephrine reuptake inhibitor (SNRI). Although some data have suggested that SNRIs can affect heart function in overdose and also may carry increased risk of death in overdose compared to selective serotonin reuptake inhibitors, their toxicity in overdose is less than that for tricyclic antidepressants.

References

Schatzberg AF, Nemeroff CB. *Textbook of psychopharmacology, fourth edition*. Washington, DC: American Psychiatric Publishing, Inc.; 2009. (Chapters 12, 18)

Stahl SM. *Stahl's essential psychopharmacology*, fourth edition. New York, NY: Cambridge University Press; 2013. (Chapter 7)

Thanacoody HK, Thomas SH. Tricyclic antidepressant poisoning: cardiovascular toxicity. *Toxicol Rev* 2005;**24**(3):205–14.

QUESTION ELEVEN

A 65-year-old patient on theophylline for chronic obstructive pulmonary disease (COPD) and fluvoxamine for recurring depressive episodes required a decreased dose of theophylline due to increased blood levels of the drug. Which of the following pharmacokinetic properties may be responsible for this?

A. Inhibition of CYP450 1A2 by fluvoxamine

B. Inhibition of CYP450 2D6 by fluvoxamine

C. Inhibition of CYP450 3A4 by fluvoxamine

Unipolar depression and antidepressants

Answer to Question Eleven

The correct answer is A.

Choice	Peer answers
A. Inhibition of CYP450 1A2 by fluvoxamine	42%
B. Inhibition of CYP450 2D6 by fluvoxamine	32%
C. Inhibition of CYP450 3A4 by fluvoxamine	26%

A Correct. Fluvoxamine is a strong inhibitor of CYP450 1A2. Theophylline is metabolized in part by CYP450 1A2, and thus strong inhibition of this enzyme by fluvoxamine may require a dose reduction of theophylline if the two are given concomitantly, so as to avoid increased blood levels of the drug.

B Incorrect. Of all SSRIs, fluvoxamine shows the least interaction with CYP450 2D6.

C Incorrect. Fluvoxamine is also a moderate inhibitor of CYP450 3A4, but since theophylline is neither a substrate nor an inhibitor of 3A4, this should not affect theophylline blood levels.

References

Schatzberg AF, Nemeroff CB. *Textbook of psychopharmacology*, fourth edition. Washington, DC: American Psychiatric Publishing, Inc.; 2009. (Chapters 13–17, 19, 21–23)

Stahl SM. *Stahl's essential psychopharmacology*, fourth edition. New York, NY: Cambridge University Press; 2013. (Chapter 7)

Stahl SM. *Stahl's essential psychopharmacology, the prescriber's guide*, fifth edition. New York, NY: Cambridge University Press; 2014.

QUESTION TWELVE

Mike is a 31-year-old patient with major depressive disorder (MDD) whose depression is responding well to the serotonin and norepinephrine reuptake inhibitor (SNRI) venlafaxine XR (150 mg/day). However, the patient acknowledges that he and his wife have been having relationship problems because of the patient's poor libido. The patient experienced this problem prior to being diagnosed and treated for MDD, but he has found that the venlafaxine has worsened this troubling symptom despite the fact that his mood has improved. Which of the following treatment strategies would you recommend for this patient?

A. Decrease venlafaxine dose

B. Switch to a norepinephrine and dopamine reuptake inhibitor (NDRI)

C. Switch to a selective serotonin reuptake inhibitor (SSRI)

D. Augment current venlafaxine dose with a phosphodiesterase-5 (e.g., sildenafil)

Unipolar depression and antidepressants

Answer to Question Twelve

The correct answer is B.

Choice	Peer answers
A. Decrease venlafaxine dose	6%
B. Switch to a norepinephrine and dopamine reuptake inhibitor (NDRI)	63%
C. Switch to a selective serotonin reuptake inhibitor (SSRI)	0%
D. Augment current venlafaxine dose with a phosphodiesterase-5 (e.g., sildenafil)	31%

The prevalence of sexual dysfunction, including diminished libido, impaired arousal, and lack of orgasm, is high among patients with MDD, and sexual dysfunction may worsen with antidepressant treatment (particularly treatment with a serotonin reuptake inhibitor). Exacerbation of sexual dysfunction by antidepressant treatment is one of the most common factors reported to cause treatment non-adherence or discontinuation.

A Incorrect. With regards to the diagnostic criteria for depression, this patient is responding well to his current dose of venlafaxine. Although lowering the dose of venlafaxine may improve this patient's sexual function, a dose reduction may also increase his risk of depressive relapse.

B Correct. Pharmacological agents that increase dopaminergic neurotransmission and/or decrease serotonergic neurotransmission are often effective in ameliorating sexual dysfunction. Switching to (or augmenting with) an NDRI such as bupropion would be expected to increase dopaminergic neurotransmission and improve sexual function.

C Incorrect. Of the available antidepressant treatments, SSRIs are associated with the greatest risk of worsening sexual function, so switching from venlafaxine to an SSRI would not be expected to improve sexual functioning.

D Incorrect. Although it is usually best to try another antidepressant monotherapy before resorting to augmentation strategies for the treatment of side effects, for a patient such as this who is otherwise responding well it might be reasonable to augment. However, phosphodiesterase-5 inhibitors do not increase desire and thus

Unipolar depression and antidepressants

would not be a good option to treat this patient's specific problems with sexual function.

References

Kennedy SH, Rizvi S. Sexual dysfunction, depression, and the impact of antidepressants. *J Clin Psychopharmacol* 2009;**29**(2):157–64.

Serretti A, Chiesa A. Sexual side effects of pharmacological treatment of psychiatric diseases. *Clin Pharmacol Ther* 2011;**89**(1):142–7.

Unipolar depression and antidepressants

QUESTION THIRTEEN

A 39-year-old patient with major depressive disorder presents to your office after several months of trying various antidepressant drugs. It is suggested that he try augmenting his current regimen with L-methylfolate. Why might L-methylfolate boost the therapeutic efficacy of antidepressants?

A. It increases synthesis of monoamines

B. It increases the release of monoamines

C. It both increases synthesis and inhibits metabolism of monoamines

Answer to Question Thirteen

The correct answer is C.

Choice	Peer answers
A. It increases synthesis of monoamines	50%
B. It increases the release of monoamines	1%
C. It both increases synthesis and inhibits metabolism of monoamines	49%

C Correct. L–methylfolate assists in the formation of a critical cofactor for the synthesis of monoamines, known as tetrahydrobiopterin, or BH4. When L–methylfolate forms the critical amount of BH4, that BH4 can activate the enzymes tyrosine hydroxylase and tryptophan hydroxylase, which synthesize the trimonoamines serotonin, norepinephrine, and dopamine. In addition, L–methylfolate could hypothetically lead to methylation of the promoter for the gene of the enzyme COMT (catechol-O-methyltransferase), which inactivates dopamine and norepinephrine. This methylation silences the gene, and decreases the synthesis of COMT enzyme, and this reduces the metabolism of dopamine and norepinephrine.

A Partially correct.

B Incorrect.

References

Schatzberg AF, Nemeroff CB. *Textbook of psychopharmacology*, fourth edition. Washington, DC: American Psychiatric Publishing, Inc.; 2009. (Chapters 62–65)

Stahl SM. Methylated spirits: epigenetic hypotheses of psychiatric disorders. *CNS Spectr* 2010;**15**(4):220–30.

Stahl SM. Fooling mother nature: epigenetics and novel treatments for psychiatric disorders. *CNS Spectr* 2010;**15**(6):358–65.

Stahl SM. *Essential psychopharmacology, the prescriber's guide*, fifth edition. New York, NY: Cambridge University Press; 2014.

Unipolar depression and antidepressants

QUESTION FOURTEEN

A 36-year-old patient has only partially responded to his second monotherapy with a first-line antidepressant. Which of the following has the best evidence of efficacy for augmenting anti-depressants in patients with inadequate response?

A. Adding an atypical antipsychotic

B. Adding buspirone

C. Adding a stimulant

Answer to Question Fourteen

The correct answer is A.

Choice	Peer answers
A. Adding an atypical antipsychotic	76%
B. Adding buspirone	13%
C. Adding a stimulant	11%

A Correct. Atypical antipsychotics have been studied as adjuncts to selective serotonin reuptake inhibitors (SSRIs) and serotonin-norepinephrine reuptake inhibitors (SNRIs), with approvals for aripiprazole, quetiapine XR, olanzapine (in combination with fluoxetine), and brexpiprazole. Overall, most studies of atypical antipsychotics show a benefit of combination treatment over mono-therapy, although effect sizes have been modest. Although atypical antipsychotics have the best evidence of efficacy for augmenting antidepressants in patients with inadequate response, their adverse event profiles may still put them later in the treatment algorithm.

B Incorrect. Although adding buspirone, a serotonin 1A partial agon-ist, to a first-line antidepressant makes sense mechanistically, the limited data that exist are mixed/weak.

C Incorrect. The limited controlled data for stimulant augmentation in depression show a trend of benefit; however, this strategy is not as well documented as is augmentation with atypical antipsychotics.

References

Bech P, Fava M, Trivedi MH, Wisniewski SR, Rush AJ. Outcomes on the pharmacopsychometric triangle in bupropion-SR vs. buspirone augmentation of citalopram in the STAR*D trial. *Acta Psychiatr Scand* 2012;**125**(4):342–8.

Citrome L. Adjunctive aripiprazole, olanzapine, or quetiapine for major depressive disorder: an analysis of number needed to treat, number needed to harm, and likelihood to be helped or harmed. *Postgrad Med* 2010;**122**(4):39–48.

Trivedi MH, Cutler, AJ, Richards C, et al. A randomized controlled trial of the efficacy and safety of lisdexamfetamine dimesylate as augmen-tation therapy in adults with residual symptoms of major depressive disorder after treatment with escitalopram. *J Clin Psychiatry* 2013;**74** (8):802–9.

Unipolar depression and antidepressants

QUESTION FIFTEEN

A 24-year-old woman suffering from a major depressive episode (moderate) presents to your office. She has previously taken an SSRI for depression but expresses a desire to try something "natural." Which of the following has the best evidence of efficacy for treating symptoms of depression?

A. Melatonin

B. Omega 3 fatty acids

C. Vitamin D

Answer to Question Fifteen

The correct answer is B.

Choice	Peer answers
A. Melatonin	13%
B. Omega 3 fatty acids	68%
C. Vitamin D	20%

A Incorrect. Recent meta-analyses of exogenous melatonin in the treatment of depression did not show any significant effect.

B Correct. Multiple meta-analyses have demonstrated modest efficacy for omega 3 fatty acids in major depressive disorder. In particular, eicosapentaenoic acid (EPA) is the effective component (vs. docosahexaenoic acid (DHA)), with 60% EPA (of total EPA+DHA) needed.

C Incorrect. Individual studies and meta-analyses have yielded mixed results regarding the efficacy of Vitamin D for treating depressive symptoms.

References

Hansen MV, Danielsen AK, Hageman I, Rosenberg J, Gogenur I. The therapeutic or prophylactic effect of exogenous melatonin against depression and depressive symptoms: A systematic review and meta-analysis. *Eur Neuropsychopharmacol* 2014 [Epub ahead of print].

Sublette ME, Ellis SP, Geant AL, Mann JJ. Meta-analysis of the effects of eicosapentaenoic acid (EPA) in clinical trials in depression. *J Clin Psychiatry* 2011;**72**(12):1577–84.

Shaffer JA, Edmondson D, Wasson LT, et al. Vitamin D supplementation for depressive symptoms: a systematic review and meta-analysis of randomized controlled trials. *Psychosom Med* 2014;**76**(3):190–6.

Spedding S. Vitamin D and depression: a systematic review and meta-analysis comparing studies with and without biological flaws. *Nutrients* 2014;**6**(4):1501–18.

Unipolar depression and antidepressants

QUESTION SIXTEEN

After being treated with sertraline for over a year, a 23-year-old man continues to suffer from significant symptoms of depressed mood and intermittent anxiety. He has recently been admitted to a substance dependence treatment program for alcohol use (up to 15 drinks per day for the last 2 years) and has been sober for 2 weeks. Psychotherapy within the program reveals that his depressed mood predated the start of his heavy drinking. There is no current suicidal ideation and no history of attempted suicide. At this point, the patient has discontinued sertraline by choice. Is he a reasonable candidate for transcranial magnetic stimulation (TMS)?

A. No; he has only had one medication trial, and at least two failed trials are required before considering TMS

B. No; there is possible alteration of consciousness due to the need for anesthesia, which would interfere with his psychotherapy

C. No; his recent alcohol dependence is a contraindication for TMS

D. Yes; he fulfills criteria to qualify for a trial of TMS

Answer to Question Sixteen

The correct answer is D.

Choice	Peer answers
A. No; he has only had one medication trial, and at least two failed trials are required before considering TMS	44%
B. No; there is possible alteration of consciousness due to the need for anesthesia, which would interfere with his psychotherapy	1%
C. No; his recent alcohol dependence is a contraindication for TMS	13%
D. Yes; he fulfills criteria to qualify for a trial of TMS	41%

TMS involves an electromagnetic coil placed on the scalp, creating a magnetic field that penetrates the skull by a few centimeters. This depolarizes neurons in the superficial cortex; through neural pathways, this local stimulation causes functional changes in other brain regions. Its approval is based on a study of high-frequency TMS over the left dorsolateral prefrontal cortex (DLPFC); however, low-frequency right-sided stimulation has also shown efficacy.

A Incorrect. TMS is approved for treatment-resistant depression, defined as having failed at least one (not two) pharmacological trials in the current episode.

B Incorrect. TMS is generally done on an outpatient basis, requires no anesthesia, and does not involve loss of consciousness.

C Incorrect. Recent alcohol dependence is not a contraindication for TMS. The only contraindication is for patients with ferromagnetic metal within 30 cm of where the electromagnetic coil is placed. Caution should be exercised for patients with an implantable device controlled by physiological signs.

D Correct.

References

Berlim MT, Van den Eynde F, Daskalakis JZ. Clinically meaningful efficacy and acceptability of low-frequency repetitive transcranial magnetic stimulation (rTMS) for treating primary major depression: a meta-analysis of randomized, double-blind and sham-controlled trials. *Neuropsychopharmacology* 2013;**38**:543–51.

Blumberger DM, Mulsant BH, Daskalakis ZJ. What is the role of brain stimulation therapies in the treatment of depression? *Curr Psychiatry Rep* 2013;**15**(7):368.

Kalu UG, Sexton CE, Loo CK, Ebmeier KP. Transcranial direct current stimulation in the treatment of major depression: a metaanalysis. *Psychological Med* 2012;**42**(9):1791–800.

O'Reardon JP, Solvason HB, Janicak PG, et al. Efficacy and safety of transcranial magnetic stimulation in the acute treatment of major depression: a multisite randomized controlled trial. *Biol Psychiatry* 2007;**62**(11):1208–16.

QUESTION SEVENTEEN

A 36-year-old woman is suffering from her third major depressive episode. She has not experienced improvement despite adequate trials of several different antidepressants and is now undergoing electroconvulsive therapy (ECT). She did not respond until the 9th session, but has now shown progressive improvement following her 10th, 11th, and 12th sessions. What would be the recommended next step for this patient?

A. Discontinue ECT and switch to a medication treatment

B. Continue ECT until she reaches a plateau of improvement, then initiate medication treatment

C. Continue ECT indefinitely (barring any significant side effects) to prevent relapse

Unipolar depression and antidepressants

Answer to Question Seventeen

The correct answer is B.

Choice	Peer answers
A. Discontinue ECT and switch to a medication treatment	11%
B. Continue ECT until she reaches a plateau of improvement, then initiate medication treatment	70%
C. Continue ECT indefinitely (barring any significant side effects) to prevent relapse	19%

B Correct. Existing data and expert clinical opinion support the idea that ECT response can be relatively rapid, often occurring after a few sessions. Consistent with this, the acute course of ECT treatment is typically 6–12 treatments and does not generally exceed 20 treatments. However, it is important that treatment continue until symptoms remit or plateau, because relapse rates are higher if ECT is discontinued prematurely.

A and C Incorrect.

References

Gelenberg AJ, Freeman MP, Markowitz JC, et al. *Practice guideline for the treatment of patients with major depressive disorder*, third edition. APA; 2010.

Husain MM, Rush AJ, Fink M, et al. Speed of response and remission in major depressive disorder with acute electroconvulsive therapy (ECT): a Consortium for Research in ECT (CORE) report. *J Clin Psychiatry* 2004;**65**(4):485–91.

Marangell LB, Martinez M, Jurdi RA, Zboyan H. Neurostimulation therapies in depression: a review of new modalities. *Acta Psychiatr Scand* 2007;**116**:174–81.

QUESTION EIGHTEEN

A 34-year-old man with depression characterized by depressed mood, sleep difficulties, and concentration problems has not responded well to a selective serotonin reuptake inhibitor (SSRI) or a serotonin-norepinephrine reuptake inhibitor. His clinician elects to switch him to vortioxetine, which has prominent 5HT7 antagonism. What may be a primary function of these receptors?

A. Regulation of serotonin–acetylcholine interactions

B. Regulation of serotonin–dopamine interactions

C. Regulation of serotonin–glutamate interactions

D. Regulation of serotonin–norepinephrine interactions

Answer to Question Eighteen

The correct answer is C.

Choice	Peer answers
A. Regulation of serotonin–acetylcholine interactions	9%
B. Regulation of serotonin–dopamine interactions	26%
C. Regulation of serotonin–glutamate interactions	58%
D. Regulation of serotonin–norepinephrine interactions	7%

C Correct. 5HT7 receptors are postsynaptic G protein-linked receptors. They are localized in the cortex, hippocampus, hypothalamus, thalamus, and brainstem raphe nuclei, where they regulate mood, circadian rhythms, sleep, learning, and memory. A major function of these receptors may be to regulate serotonin-glutamate interactions.

Serotonin can both activate and inhibit glutamate release from cortical pyramidal neurons. Serotonin released from neurons in the raphe nucleus can bind to 5HT2A receptors on pyramidal glutamate neurons in the prefrontal cortex, activating glutamate release. However, serotonin also binds to 5HT1A receptors on pyramidal glutamate neurons, an action that inhibits glutamate release. Additionally, serotonin binds to 5HT7 receptors on GABA interneurons in the prefrontal cortex. This stimulates GABA release, which in turn inhibits glutamate release.

Serotonin binding at 5HT7 receptors can also inhibit its own release. That is, when serotonergic neurons in the raphe nucleus are stimulated, they release serotonin throughout the brain, including not only in the prefrontal cortex but also in the raphe nucleus itself. Serotonin can then bind to 5HT7 receptors on GABA interneurons in the raphe nucleus. This stimulates GABA release, which then turns off serotonin release.

Serotonin binding at 5HT7 receptors in the raphe nucleus inhibits serotonin release; therefore, an antagonist at this receptor would be expected to enhance serotonin release. Specifically, by blocking serotonin from binding to the 5HT7 receptor on GABA interneurons, a 5HT7 antagonist would prevent the release of GABA onto serotonin neurons, thus allowing the continued release of serotonin in the prefrontal cortex.

A, B, and D Incorrect.

References

Sarkisyan G, Roberts AJ, Hedlund PB. The 5-HT7 receptor as a mediator and modulator of antidepressant-like behavior. *Behav Brain Res* 2010;**209**(1):99–108.

Stahl SM. The serotonin-7 receptor as a novel therapeutic target. *J Clin Psychiatry* 2010;**71**(11):1414–5.

Unipolar depression and antidepressants

QUESTION NINETEEN

A 32-year-old woman with major depressive disorder has been taking a selective serotonin reuptake inhibitor (SSRI) with good response for 9 months. She presents now with complaints that she feels numb, and that even when she's sad she can't cry. Her clinician is considering reducing the dose of her SSRI in an effort to alleviate this problem. Is this a reasonable option?

A. Yes, data suggest that SSRI-induced indifference is dose-dependent and can be alleviated by reducing the dose

B. No, although data suggest that SSRI-induced indifference is dose-dependent, patients who develop this side effect generally require switch to a different medication

C. No, SSRI-induced indifference is not dose-dependent and thus cannot be alleviated by reducing the dose

Answer to Question Nineteen

The correct answer is A.

Choice	Peer answers
A. Yes, data suggest that SSRI-induced indifference is dose-dependent and can be alleviated by reducing the dose	70%
B. No, although data suggest that SSRI-induced indifference is dose-dependent, patients who develop this side effect generally require switch to a different medication	25%
C. No, SSRI-induced indifference is not dose-dependent and thus cannot be alleviated by reducing the dose	5%

A Correct. Apathy and emotional blunting can be symptoms of depression, but they are also side effects associated with selective serotonin reuptake inhibitors (SSRIs). These symptoms − termed "SSRI-induced indifference" − are under-recognized but can be very distressing for patients. They are theoretically due to an increase in serotonin levels and a consequent reduction of dopamine release. The first recommended strategy for addressing SSRI-induced indifference is to lower the SSRI dose, if feasible. Additional options include adding an augmenting agent, or switching to an antidepressant in another class.

B and C Incorrect.

References
Sansone RA, Sansone LA. SSRI-induced indifference. *Psychiatry (Edgemont)* 2010;**7**(1):14–8.

Stahl SM. *Case studies: Stahl's essential psychopharmacology.* New York, NY: Cambridge University Press; 2011.

Stahl SM. *Stahl's essential psychopharmacology*, fourth edition. New York, NY: Cambridge University Press; 2013. (Chapter 7)

Stahl SM. *Stahl's essential psychopharmacology, the prescriber's guide*, fifth edition. New York, NY: Cambridge University Press; 2014.

Unipolar depression and antidepressants

QUESTION TWENTY

A 36-year-old woman with longstanding depression is currently experiencing a severe episode characterized by depressed mood, hypersomnia, lack of pleasure, and suicidality. She has not responded to multiple medication trials, including first-line agents, augmentation strategies, and a monoamine oxidase inhibitor. She has also failed to respond to electroconvulsive therapy. Her treatment team is now considering ketamine. This is based on a current leading hypothesis that posits that depression may be related to:

A. Glutamate hypoactivity

B. Glutamate hyperactivity

C. NMDA receptor hypofunctioning

D. NMDA receptor hyperfunctioning

Answer to Question Twenty

The correct answer is B.

Choice	Peer answers
A. Glutamate hypoactivity	11%
B. Glutamate hyperactivity	44%
C. NMDA receptor hypofunctioning	35%
D. NMDA receptor hyperfunctioning	10%

B Correct. As evidenced by studies with ketamine, an NMDA receptor antagonist can have rapid antidepressant effects by reducing glutamate activity and thus compensating for glutamate hyperactivity.

A Incorrect. The leading hypothesis of depression is glutamate hyperactivity, not hypoactivity.

C Incorrect. Ketamine is an NMDA blocker and has been shown to improve depression and suicidality in the short term (i.e., for a few days). Many other agents being investigated in treatment-resistant depression are also anti-glutamatergic but have different mechanisms than NMDA blockade. Thus, the leading hypothesis regarding glutamate in depression is glutamate hyperactivity in general; the hypothesis is not specifically related to NMDA receptor functioning.

D Incorrect (NMDA receptor hyperfunctioning).

References
Stahl SM. *Stahl's essential psychopharmacology*, fourth edition. New York, NY: Cambridge University Press; 2013. (Chapter 7)

Zarate CA Jr, Singh JB, Carlson PJ, et al. A randomized trial of an N-methyl-D-aspartate antagonist in treatment-resistant major depression. *Arch Gen Psychiatry* 2006;**63**:856–64.

Unipolar depression and antidepressants

QUESTION TWENTY ONE

A 24-year-old woman with depression has just had genetic testing, including testing of the genes for catechol-O-methyltransferase (COMT) and methylenetetrahydrofolate reductase (MTHFR). Her symptoms are theoretically consistent with severe dopamine deficiency with apathy, anhedonia, psychomotor retardation, and cognitive slowing. Based on current literature, what genetic testing results might be most likely?

A. COMT Val/Val and MTHFR (T/T) or (C/T)

B. COMT Val/Val and MTHFR (C/C)

C. COMT Met/Met and MTHFR (T/T) or (C/T)

D. COMT Met/Met and MTHFR (C/C)

Answer to Question Twenty One

The correct answer is A.

Choice	Peer answers
A. COMT Val/Val and MTHFR (T/T) or (C/T)	53%
B. COMT Val/Val and MTHFR (C/C)	15%
C. COMT Met/Met and MTHFR (T/T) or (C/T)	25%
D. COMT Met/Met and MTHFR (C/C)	6%

The COMT gene contains a highly functional and common variation (position 472, guanine to adenine substitution) that causes a valine to methionine change in peptide sequence of COMT enzyme at codon 108/158 (val108/158 met). This results in COMT enzyme activity that is significantly reduced:

Allele	Met/Met	Met/Val	Val/Val
Activity	low	intermediate	high

The prefrontal cortex has few dopamine transporters; thus, dopamine inactivation in the prefrontal cortex is more dependent upon COMT metabolism. Therefore when COMT activity is high (as with COMT158 Val) there is decreased dopamine in the prefrontal cortex, which in turn can be associated with cognitive deficits.

MTHFR is the predominant enzyme that converts inactive folic acid to an active form of folate. The 677 T allele is associated with decreased MTHFR activity, leading to increased homocysteine and decreased methylation capacity. This can increase expression of COMT and lead to reduced dopamine.

Decreased methylation of COMT, caused by decreased function with the MTHFR 677T variant, hypothetically results in decreased dopamine signaling and may ultimately lead to cognitive impairments. This effect could hypothetically be exacerbated in patients who carry both the MTHFR 677T allele and the high–activity COMT 158 Val/Val genotype, with increased cognitive impairment. This effect has been demonstrated in schizophrenic patients but not in healthy controls.

A Correct. Carrying both the COMT 158 Val/Val and the MTHFR 677 (T/T) or (C/T) genotypes theoretically would result in increased degradation of dopamine in the prefrontal cortex, leading to decreased dopamine signaling and associated cognitive dysfunction, apathy, and psychomotor retardation ("prefrontal dopamine" hypothesis).

B Incorrect. COMT158 Val/Val would theoretically result in decreased dopamine; however, MTHFR (C/C) would not.

C Incorrect. COMT158 Met/Met would theoretically result in *decreased* degradation of dopamine, and thus *increased* dopamine signaling.

D Incorrect.

References

Baune B, Hohoff C, Berger K, et al. Association of the COMT val158-met variant with antidepressant treatment response in major depression. *Neuropsychopharmacology* 2008;**33**:924–32.

Kato M, Serretti A. Review and meta-analysis of antidepressant pharmacogenetic findings in major depressive disorder. *Mol Psychiatry* 2010;**15**:473–500.

Kirchheiner J, Nickchen K, Bauer M, et al. Pharmacogenetics of antidepressants and antipsychotics: the contribution of allelic variations to the phenotype of drug response. *Mol Psychiatry* 2004;**9**:442–73.

Kocabas NA, Faghel C, Barreto M, et al. The impact of catechol-O-methyltransferase SNPs and haplotypes on treatment response phenotypes in major depressive disorder: a case-control association study. *Int Clin Psychopharmacol* 2010;**25**(4):218–27.

Nutt D, Demyttenaere K, Janka Z, et al. The other face of depression, reduced positive affect: the role of catecholamines in causation and cure. *J Psychopharmacol* 2006;**21**(5):461–71.

QUESTION TWENTY TWO

The labels for antidepressants (SSRIs in particular) include several warning statements about possible adverse effects of use during pregnancy. Which of the following has the most evidence suggesting an increased risk with antidepressant use during pregnancy?

A. First trimester cardiac malformations

B. Persistent pulmonary hypertension of the newborn (PPHN)

C. Postnatal adaptation syndrome (PNAS)

D. Long-term neurodevelopmental abnormalities

Answer to Question Twenty Two

The correct answer is C.

Choice	Peer answers
A. First trimester cardiac malformations	19%
B. Persistent pulmonary hypertension of the newborn (PPHN)	28%
C. Postnatal adaptation syndrome (PNAS)	49%
D. Long-term neurodevelopmental abnormalities	4%

A Incorrect. The evidence for increased risk of first trimester major malformations with antidepressants has been limited and inconsistent. Paroxetine, which carries a warning and a Pregnancy Risk Category of D, has shown increased risk of major and cardiac malformations in several studies, although this has not been seen in large database assessments. Limited data with bupropion has also shown possible increased risk of congenital heart defects. The results of these studies suggest that any increase in the absolute risk of cardiac malformations with antidepressant use is small. Consistent with this, a recent large, population-based cohort study did not identify a substantial increase in risk of cardiac malformations (relative risk vs. women with untreated depression was 1.06).

B Incorrect. Persistent pulmonary hypertension of the newborn (PPHN) is a rare condition with a baseline risk of 1.9 per 1000 live births. Nonetheless, PPHN is fatal in approximately 20% of cases and is thus a serious concern. A recent meta-analysis has shown that although antidepressant (SSRI) use in late pregnancy does increase the risk for PPHN, the absolute risk remains small (4.75–5.40 per 1000 live births). The number needed to harm (NNH) in the meta-analysis was 286–351 – in other words, an additional 286 to 351 women would need to be treated with an SSRI in late pregnancy in order for one additional case of PPHN to occur.

C Correct. Postnatal adaptation syndrome (PNAS) in infants is characterized by irritability, abnormal crying, tremor, lethargy, hypoactivity, decreased feeding, tachypnea, and respiratory distress. Although there is some conflicting evidence, overall, data suggest that PNAS can occur in 20–30% of infants exposed to serotonergic antidepressants. PNAS has most often been reported with paroxetine, fluoxetine, or venlafaxine, but could theoretically occur with any antidepressant.

D Incorrect. The data regarding the risk of long-term neurodevelopmental abnormalities with prenatal antidepressants are very limited. No studies have found detrimental effects on cognitive development. Two studies have found possible effects on motor developments. Overall, the existing studies are reassuring but have limitations: most do not follow children through school age, control for maternal IQ, or measure maternal treatment adherence.

References

Byatt N, Deligiannidis KM, Freeman MP. Antidepressant use in pregnancy: a critical review focused on risks and controversies. *Acta Psychiatr Scand* 2013;**127**:94–114.

Gentile S, Galbally M. Prenatal exposure to antidepressant medications and neurodevelopmental outcomes: a systematic review. *J Affective Disord* 2011;**128**:1–9.

Grigoriadis S, Vonderporten EH, Mamisashvili L, et al. Prenatal exposure to antidepressants and persistent pulmonary hypertension of the newborn: systematic review and meta-analysis. *BMJ* 2014;348:**f6932**.

Huybrechts KF, Palmsten K, Avorn J, et al. Antidepressant use in pregnancy and the risk of cardiac defects. *N Engl J Med* 2014;**370** (25):2397–407.

QUESTION TWENTY THREE

Sasha is a 58-year-old patient with a history of depression who has been prescribed agomelatine. At present, she is relatively free of depressive symptoms, likely due in part to binding of agomelatine to what receptors in the suprachiasmatic nucleus?

A. Melatonin receptors

B. Serotonin 2C receptors

C. Melatonin and serotonin 2C receptors

Answer to Question Twenty Three

The correct answer is C.

Choice	Peer answers
A. Melatonin receptors	19%
B. Serotonin 2C receptors	14%
C. Melatonin and serotonin 2C receptors	67%

A and B Partially correct.

C Correct. Agomelatine is both a melatonin M1 and M2 receptor agonist and a serotonin 5HT2C receptor antagonist. This unique receptor profile gives agomelatine the ability to address impairments in neurotransmission as well as circadian rhythm dysfunction. First, agomelatine can modulate circadian rhythms through its agonist actions at melatonin receptors. Melatonin is normally released from the pineal gland in response to environmental cues. It then acts on the suprachiasmatic nucleus, the location of the master clock, to reset circadian rhythms. Thus, as an agonist at melatonin receptors, agomelatine likewise regulates the molecular clock and can resynchronize circadian rhythms that are disturbed in depression.

Second, agomelatine affects neurotransmission by blocking 5HT2C receptors. Normally, serotonin excites GABA interneurons by stimulating 5HT2C receptors, which increases the release of the inhibitory neurotransmitter GABA. GABA can then bind to $GABA_A$ receptors on noradrenergic and dopaminergic neurons, Since GABA is inhibitory, it will prevent these neurons from releasing norepinephrine and dopamine in the prefrontal cortex. As a 5HT2C receptor antagonist, agomelatine blocks serotonin from binding to GABA interneurons. This leads to disinhibition of monoaminergic neurons and increased norepinephrine and dopamine in the prefrontal cortex, which could potentially improve mood and cognition.

References
DeBodinat C, Guardiola-Lemaitre B, Mocaer E, et al. Agomelatine, the first melatonergic antidepressant: discovery, characterization, and development. *Nature Reviews Drug Discovery* 2010;**9**:628–42.

Chapter peer comparison

For the Unipolar depression and antidepressants section, the correct answer was selected 62% of the time.

4 BIPOLAR DISORDER AND MOOD STABILIZERS

QUESTION ONE

A 34-year-old man has recently been diagnosed with bipolar disorder, 6 years after his symptoms began. He has had no mood stabilizing treatment in that time. According to the kindling model and allostatic load hypothesis, what progressive pattern of illness would you expect this patient to have exhibited over the course of the last 6 years?

A. Longer interval between episodes, worsened emotionality, minimal change in cognitive impairment

B. Shorter interval between episodes, worsened emotionality, minimal change in cognitive impairment

C. Longer interval between episodes, worsened emotionality, worsened cognitive impairment

D. Shorter interval between episodes, worsened emotionality, worsened cognitive impairment

Answer to Question One

The correct answer is D.

Choice	Peer answers
A. Longer interval between episodes, worsened emotionality, minimal change in cognitive impairment	3%
B. Shorter interval between episodes, worsened emotionality, minimal change in cognitive impairment	19%
C. Longer interval between episodes, worsened emotionality, worsened cognitive impairment	1%
D. Shorter interval between episodes, worsened emotionality, worsened cognitive impairment	77%

A, B, and C Incorrect.

D Correct. Throughout the course of illness, patients with bipolar disorder will experience manic or hypomanic episodes, depressive episodes, and inter-episode periods during which they are generally well but may have subsyndromal symptoms. The pattern of episodes can differ for each patient; however, in general the clinical course of bipolar disorder is progressive. That is, as the number of episodes a person has had increases, the **interval between episodes gets shorter** and **emotionality may worsen**. In addition, **cognitive impairment seems to worsen** with the length of illness. Increasing episode number is also associated with reduced likelihood of treatment response.

Models for how these changes may come to be posit that recurrent mood episodes are associated with repeated physiological insults that add up and kindle, like a spark bursting into fire. This could compromise endogenous compensatory mechanisms, leading to cell apoptosis that in turn causes rewiring of the brain circuits involved in mood regulation and cognition. This can render one more vulnerable to the effects of stressors, increasing risk of future episodes and thus perpetuating the vicious spiral.

References
Berk M, Kapczinski F, Andreazza AC, et al. Pathways underlying neuroprogression in bipolar disorder: focus on inflammation, oxidative stress, and neurotrophic factors. *Neurosci Biobeh Rev* 2011;**35**(3):804–17.

Bipolar disorder and mood stabilizers

Kapczinksi F, Vieta E, Andreazza AC, et al. Allostatic load in bipolar disorder: implications for pathophysiology and treatment. *Neurosci Biobeh Rev* 2008;**32**:675–92.

Post RM. Kindling and sensitization as models for affective episode recurrence, cyclicity, and tolerance phenomena. *Neurosci Biobeh Rev* 2007;**31**:858–73.

QUESTION TWO

A 28-year-old woman with bipolar disorder recently began taking a mood stabilizer and has experienced improvement in her symptoms. Which of the following are mechanisms by which different mood stabilizers may prevent mitochondrial dysfunction in bipolar disorder?

A. Increasing levels of anti–apoptotic proteins

B. Decreasing levels of pro–apoptotic proteins

C. Increasing levels of key antioxidants

D. A and B

E. A, B, and C

Bipolar disorder and mood stabilizers

Answer to Question Two

The correct answer is E.

Choice	Peer answers
A. Increasing levels of anti-apoptotic proteins	6%
B. Decreasing levels of pro-apoptotic proteins	9%
C. Increasing levels of key antioxidants	4%
D. A and B	20%
E. A, B, and C	60%

Mitochondria are intracellular organelles that regulate energy through cell respiration. They also play critical roles in regulating cell apoptosis. Mitochondrial dysfunction can therefore contribute to inappropriate cell damage and death.

There are multiple ways in which mitochondrial dysfunction can lead to apoptosis. Mitochondria contain both pro- and anti-apoptotic proteins that must remain in a delicate balance to control the integrity of the mitochondrial membrane. If that balance is shifted, this can cause morphological changes to the mitochondrial membrane, allowing the release of cytochrome C and other substances that induce apoptosis.

One factor that may shift the balance of pro- and anti-apoptotic proteins is an excess of free radicals, which themselves are produced by mitochondria during cell respiration. Normally, antioxidant defenses in the brain can stabilize the free radicals, thus creating oxidative balance. If antioxidants are depleted, then free radicals may accumulate and activate pro-apoptotic proteins, thus initiating the mitochondrial pathway of apoptosis.

E Correct. Both lithium and valproate have been shown to **increase levels of the anti-apoptotic protein** Bcl-2, thus maintaining the balance of pro- and anti-apoptotic proteins, restoring the integrity of the mitochondrial membrane, and preventing release of cytochrome C. Some atypical antipsychotics may **reduce elevated levels of the pro-apoptotic protein Bax**. Lithium and valproate have both been shown **to increase levels of the antioxidant glutathione**, which may help reduce the presence of free radicals and thus prevent activation of the mitochondrial pathway of apoptosis.

A, B, C, and D Incorrect.

References
Bachman RF, Wang Y, Yuan P, et al. Common effects of lithium and valproate on mitochondrial functions: protection against

methamphetamine-induced mitochondrial damage. *Int J Neuropsychopharmacol* 2009;**12**:805–22.

Berk M, Kapczinski F, Andreazza AC, et al. Pathways underlying neuroprogression in bipolar disorder: focus on inflammation, oxidative stress, and neurotrophic factors. *Neurosci Biobeh Rev* 2011;**35**(3):804–17.

Hunsberger J, Austin DR, Henter ID, Chen G. The neurotrophic and neuroprotective effects of psychotropic agents. *Dialogues Clin Neurosci* 2009;**11**(3):333–48.

Bipolar disorder and mood stabilizers

QUESTION THREE

A 23-year-old female presents complaining that her short temper has lost her important friendships and other relationships. She has already gotten in significant trouble in the dorms in college, stealing a fire extinguisher, driving on the common area lawn, and hostilely addressing a professor. Which of the following monoamine projections may account for her recent behavior? Projections to the:

A. Ventromedial prefrontal cortex

B. Orbital frontal cortex

C. Striatum

D. A and B

E. A and C

F. B and C

Answer to Question Three

The correct answer is D.

Choice	Peer answers
A. Ventromedial prefrontal cortex	15%
B. Orbital frontal cortex	11%
C. Striatum	1%
D. A and B	54%
E. A and C	11%
F. B and C	7%

D   Correct, as A and B are correct. Projections of all three monoamines to the **ventromedial prefrontal cortex** are thought to be associated with symptoms of mania such as **irritable mood**. Projections of all three monoamines to the **orbital frontal cortex** are thought to be associated with symptoms of mania, such as **risk taking** and **impulsive control**.

C   Incorrect. Dopaminergic and serotonergic projections to **the striatum** are thought to be associated with symptoms of mania, such as increased **goal-directed activity** or **agitation**.

E and F   Incorrect.

References

Schatzberg AF, Nemeroff CB. *Textbook of psychopharmacology*, fourth edition. Washington, DC: American Psychiatric Publishing, Inc.; 2009. (Chapter 45)

Stahl SM. *Stahl's essential psychopharmacology*, fourth edition. New York, NY: Cambridge University Press; 2013. (Chapter 8)

Bipolar disorder and mood stabilizers

QUESTION FOUR

A 32-year-old woman with bipolar I disorder has just found out that she is 6 weeks pregnant. Her mania has been stable on a combination of lithium, valproate, and quetiapine, but she is unsure about the safety of maintaining her medications during her pregnancy. Which of the following is true regarding the use of these medications for bipolar disorder during pregnancy?

A. Lithium has known teratogenic effects and is not a preferred treatment

B. Lithium and valproate have known teratogenic effects and are not preferred treatments

C. Lithium, valproate, and quetiapine have known teratogenic effects and are not preferred treatments

Answer to Question Four

The correct answer is B.

Choice	Peer answers
A. Lithium has known teratogenic effects and is not a preferred treatment	4%
B. Lithium and valproate have known teratogenic effects and are not preferred treatments	83%
C. Lithium, valproate, and quetiapine have known teratogenic effects and are not preferred treatments	13%

A Incorrect. Lithium has known teratogenic effects, but so does valproate.

B Correct. Both lithium and valproate have known teratogenic effects. Lithium is Pregnancy Risk Category D and has evidence of increased risk of major birth defects and cardiac anomalies, especially Ebstein's anomaly, although a recent review suggested that the risk of cardiac anomalies may be over-emphasized. Valproate is also Pregnancy Risk Category D, with increased risk of neural tube defects (e.g., spina bifida) and other congenital anomalies.

C Incorrect. Quetiapine does not have known teratogenic effects. It is currently Pregnancy Risk Category C. If quetiapine or another atypical antipsychotic is used during pregnancy, weight gain and the risk for gestational diabetes should be more carefully monitored, with glucose tolerance testing (as opposed to glucose challenge testing) at 14–16 weeks and again at 28 weeks. After delivery, infants should be monitored for neonatal withdrawal, toxicity, extrapyramidal side effects (EPS), and sedation.

References

Galbally M, Snellen M, Power J. Antipsychotic drugs in pregnancy: a review of their maternal and fetal effects. *Therapeutic Adv Drug Safety* 2014;**5**(2):100–9;

Gentile S. Antipsychotic therapy during early and late pregnancy. A systematic review. *Schizophr Bull* 2010;**36**(3):518–44.

Stahl SM. *Stahl's essential psychopharmacology: the prescriber's guide*, fifth edition. New York, NY: Cambridge University Press; 2014.

Yacobi S, Ornoy A. Is lithium a real teratogen? What can we conclude from the prospective versus retrospective studies? A review. *Isr J Psychiatry Relat Sci* 2008;**45**(2):95–106.

Bipolar disorder and mood stabilizers

QUESTION FIVE

A 28-year-old woman presents with a depressive episode. She has previously been hospitalized and treated for a manic episode but is not currently taking any medication. The agents with the strongest evidence of efficacy in bipolar depression are:

A. Lamotrigine, lithium, quetiapine

B. Quetiapine, olanzapine–fluoxetine, lurasidone

C. Olanzapine–fluoxetine, lurasidone, lamotrigine

D. Lurasidone, lamotrigine, lithium

Answer to Question Five

The correct answer is B.

Choice	Peer answers
A. Lamotrigine, lithium, quetiapine	22%
B. Quetiapine, olanzapine-fluoxetine, lurasidone	58%
C. Olanzapine-fluoxetine, lurasidone, lamotrigine	15%
D. Lurasidone, lamotrigine, lithium	5%

A Incorrect. Controlled data assessing the efficacy of lithium in bipolar depression are too limited to draw conclusions; empiric evidence suggests that this agent may not be as effective in the depressed phase as in the manic phase or for maintenance treatment. Lithium does have evidence for reducing suicidality, however. Lamotrigine has been tested in more trials than lithium, but a recent meta-analysis failed to support its efficacy.

B Correct. Quetiapine, olanzapine–fluoxetine, and lurasidone have all demonstrated consistent efficacy in bipolar depression and are approved for this stage of the disorder.

Drug	Daily dose
Lurasidone	20–120 mg
Olanzapine-fluoxetine	6–12/25–50 mg
Quetiapine	300 mg

C Incorrect. Consistent evidence of efficacy does not exist for lamotrigine.

D Incorrect. Consistent evidence of efficacy does not exist for lamotrigine or lithium.

References

Nivoli AMA, Colom F, Murru A, et al. New treatment guidelines for acute bipolar depression. A systematic review. *J Aff Disord* 2010;**129**:14–26.

Selle V, Schalkwijk S, Vazquez GH, Baldessarini RJ. Treatments for acute bipolar depression: meta-analyses of placebo-controlled, monotherapy trials of anticonvulsants, lithium and antipsychotics. *Pharmacopsychiatry* 2014;**47**(2):43–52.

Bipolar disorder and mood stabilizers

QUESTION SIX

A 24-year-old female patient, who recently moved from Germany, presents to your office during a manic episode that initiated following abrupt discontinuation of her medication as she ran out of her prescription. She informs you that she had been diagnosed with rapid-cycling bipolar disorder, and wants to be prescribed the same medication she used to take in Germany but does not remember the generic name of the medication. She gives you the following information: she was on 1250 mg/day; she gained weight when she started it, which she did not like, but she liked the sedating effects of the drug, which helped calm her down and sleep at night. Her German doctor had told her she could experience the following side effects: hair loss, hepatotoxicity, and seizure upon abrupt withdrawal. Also she knows that she should consider switching medications when she intends to become pregnant, as the medication can lead to birth defects. Which medication was she most probably taking?

A. Lamotrigine

B. Gabapentin

C. Aripiprazole

D. Valproate

Answer to Question Six

The correct answer is D.

Choice	Peer answers
A. Lamotrigine	0%
B. Gabapentin	0%
C. Aripiprazole	0%
D. Valproate	100%

A   Incorrect. The dose range of **lamotrigine** is 100–200 mg/day, and lamotrigine does not generally induce sedation or weight gain, thus this is not the correct answer. Patients with epilepsy could seize upon abrupt discontinuation of lamotrigine, but this medication has no known teratogenic side effects and does not induce hepatotoxicity or hair loss. Lamotrigine seems to be more effective in treating depressive episodes than manic episodes in bipolar disorder.

B   Incorrect. The dose range of **gabapentin** is 900–1800 mg/day, and this medication does induce sedation, and upon rapid discontinuation it can lead to relapses in bipolar patients. However, hepatotoxicity is unusual with gabapentin, as is hair loss. Gabapentin is not known to be efficacious for bipolar disorder.

C   Incorrect. The dose range of **aripiprazole** is 15–30 mg/day. Additionally, aripiprazole does not normally induce weight gain or sedation, and has no known teratogenic effects.

D   Correct. **Valproate** is one of the first-line treatments for rapid-cycling bipolar disorder, and can induce all the side effects mentioned by the patient. The dose range is 1200–1500 mg/day for mania, and rapid discontinuation increases the risk of relapse.

References

Schatzberg AF, Nemeroff CB. *Textbook of psychopharmacology*, fourth edition. Washington, DC: American Psychiatric Publishing, Inc.; 2009. (Chapters 36–40)

Stahl SM. *Stahl's essential psychopharmacology*, fourth edition. New York, NY: Cambridge University Press; 2013. (Chapter 8)

Stahl SM. *Essential psychopharmacology, the prescriber's guide*, fifth edition. New York, NY: Cambridge University Press; 2014.

Bipolar disorder and mood stabilizers

QUESTION SEVEN

A 17-year-old girl presents with symptoms of depression. She has always been a good student and a caring and responsible sister to her two younger siblings. Recently, she has become somewhat withdrawn and reports feeling sad much of the time. Her MADRS score is 29, indicating moderate depression. This patient has also gained a significant amount of weight over the past several months, is irritable, and endorses hypersomnia. There is no information regarding family history, as the patient is adopted. Although not definitive, this particular symptom profile may be more suggestive of:

A. Unipolar depression

B. Bipolar depression

Answer to Question Seven

The correct answer is B.

Choice	Peer answers
A. Unipolar depression	42%
B. Bipolar depression	58%

A Incorrect. Data to date suggest that, although in no way definitive, there may be certain symptoms and course-related factors that help differentiate between unipolar and bipolar depression. This patient's presentation, which includes hypersomnia, weight gain, and early onset, raises the suspicion that this may be part of a bipolar illness rather than a unipolar illness.

B Correct. The patient's presentation includes multiple factors that may be more likely to occur with bipolar disorder rather than with unipolar depression. This is not definitive but does suggest caution when making treatment decisions. Although also not definitive, family history and input from someone close to the patient are generally more valuable than specific symptoms.

Suspect bipolar depression if:	Suspect unipolar depression if:
Hypersomnia and/or increased napping	Initial insomnia/ reduced sleep
Hyperphagia and/or weight gain	Appetite loss and/or weight loss
Other atypical depressive symptoms (e.g., leaden paralysis)	
Psychomotor retardation	Normal or increased activity level
Psychotic features and/or pathological guilt	Somatic complaints
Mood lability	
Early onset of first depression (25 years?)	Later onset of first depression (> 25 years?)
Multiple prior episodes (> 4?)	
	Long duration of current episode (> 6 months?)

(cont.)

Suspect bipolar depression if:	Suspect unipolar depression if:
Positive family history of bipolar disorder	Negative family history of bipolar disorder
Substance-induced mood symptoms do not resolve with discontinuation of the inciting agent, but instead require treatment with mood stabilizers	

References
Benazzi F. A continuity between bipolar II depression and major depressive disorder? *Prog Neuropsychopharmacol Biol Psychiatry* 2006;**30**:1043–50.
Motovsky B, Pecenak J. Psychopathological characteristics of bipolar and unipolar depression – potential indicators of bipolarity. *Psychiatr Danub* 2013;**25**(1):34–9.
Stahl SM. Controversies in treating bipolar depression. *CNS Spectrums* 2013;**18**(4):175–6.

QUESTION EIGHT

The "bipolar storm" refers to the concept that unstable, unregulated, and excessive neurotransmission occurs at synapses in specific brain regions, and both voltage-sensitive sodium channels and voltage-sensitive calcium channels are involved in this excessive stimulation of glutamate release. Which drugs would theoretically reduce glutamate release by blocking voltage-sensitive sodium channels?

A. Valproate and lamotrigine

B. Pregabalin and gabapentin

C. Levetiracetam and amantadine

Answer to Question Eight

The correct answer is A.

Choice	Peer answers
A. Valproate and lamotrigine	89%
B. Pregabalin and gabapentin	8%
C. Levetiracetam and amantadine	3%

A Correct. **Valproate** is a nonspecific voltage-sensitive sodium channel modulator and **lamotrigine** also blocks voltage-sensitive sodium channels, hypothesized to lead to reduction in glutamate release.

B Incorrect. **Pregabalin** and **gabapentin** are alpha 2 delta ligands at voltage-sensitive calcium channels, which also lead to reduction in glutamate release.

C Incorrect. **Levetiracetam** is a modulator of the synaptic vesicle protein SV2A, and **amantadine** is an antagonist of the NDMA receptor. While this combination of drugs would lead to reduced glutamate release, it would not do so via the mechanisms of action asked.

References

Schatzberg AF, Nemeroff CB. *Textbook of psychopharmacology*, fourth edition. Washington, DC: American Psychiatric Publishing, Inc.; 2009. (Chapters 36–40)

Sitges M, Chiu LM, Guarneros A, Nekrassov V. Effects of carbamazepine, phenytoin, lamotrigine, oxcarbazepine, topiramate, and vinpocetine on NA+ channel-mediated release of [3H]glutamate in hippocampal nerve endings. *Neuropharmacology* 2007;**52**(2):598–605.

Stahl SM. *Stahl's essential psychopharmacology*, third edition. New York, NY: Cambridge University Press; 2008. (Chapters 5, 13)

QUESTION NINE

Janet is a 43-year-old patient with bipolar disorder. She is currently depressed with some features of hypomania. Practice guidelines from the International Society for Bipolar Disorders (ISBD) recommend treatment with an antidepressant in patients with bipolar disorder under the following conditions:

A. As adjunct for acute bipolar I or II depressive episode with ≥ 2 concomitant manic symptoms, psychomotor agitation, or rapid cycling

B. As adjunct during manic and depressive episodes with mixed features

C. As adjunct in patients with predominantly mixed states

D. All of the above

E. None of the above

Answer to Question Nine

The correct answer is E.

Choice	Peer answers
A. As adjunct for acute bipolar I or II depressive episode with ≥ 2 concomitant manic symptoms, psychomotor agitation, or rapid cycling	7%
B. As adjunct during manic and depressive episodes with mixed features	3%
C. As adjunct in patients with predominantly mixed states	9%
D. All of the above	5%
E. None of the above	76%

While acknowledging the controversies and limited data surrounding the use of antidepressants in bipolar disorder, the International Society for Bipolar Disorders (ISBD) recently released recommendations related to their use. In general, the ISBD does not recommend antidepressant monotherapy in bipolar illness. Recommendations for adjunct use of antidepressants are explained below.

A Incorrect. The ISBD does not recommend using adjunct antidepressants in patients with acute bipolar I or II depressive episode and at least two concomitant manic symptoms, psychomotor agitation, or rapid cycling. However, the ISBD states that adjunct antidepressants may be considered in patients with acute bipolar I or II depression in the absence of the above-mentioned symptoms if the patient has a history of positive response to antidepressants.

B Incorrect. The ISBD does not recommend using antidepressants in patients with manic or depressive episodes with mixed features.

C Incorrect. The ISBD does not recommend using antidepressants in patients with predominantly mixed states.

D Incorrect (all of the above).

E Correct (none of the above).

References
10th International Conference on Bipolar Disorders (ICBD). Abstract 13. 2013.

QUESTION TEN

A 24-year-old woman with no history of psychiatric symptoms presents with a major depressive episode and is prescribed an antidepressant. She quickly experiences improved mood and exhibits symptoms suggestive of hypomania. Recommendations from the International Society for Bipolar Disorders (ISBD) state that the patient's antidepressant should be:

A. Discontinued

B. Maintained, but ONLY IF a mood stabilizer is added

Bipolar disorder and mood stabilizers

Answer to Question Ten

The correct answer is A.

Choice	Peer answers
A. Discontinued	72%
B. Maintained, but ONLY IF a mood stabilizer is added	28%

A Correct. The ISBD does not recommend maintaining an antidepressant if patient shows signs of (hypo)mania or increased psychomotor agitation during antidepressant treatment.

B Incorrect.

References
10th International Conference on Bipolar Disorders (ICBD). Abstract 13. 2013.

QUESTION ELEVEN

A 24-year-old man has been taking lithium for 3 years to treat his bipolar disorder. What are two primary candidates for the direct mechanisms of lithium?

A. Inhibition of glycogen synthase kinase 3β (GSK-3β) and inositol monophosphatase (IMPase)

B. Activation of GSK-3β and IMPase

C. Inhibition of GSK-3β and activation of IMPase

D. Activation of GSK-3β and inhibition of IMPase

Answer to Question Eleven

The correct answer is A.

Choice	Peer answers
A. Inhibition of glycogen synthase kinase 3β (GSK-3β) and inositol monophosphatase (IMPase)	59%
B. Activation of GSK-3β and IMPase	9%
C. Inhibition of GSK-3β and activation of IMPase	23%
D. Activation of GSK-3β and inhibition of IMPase	10%

A Correct. Lithium has been a first-line treatment for bipolar disorder for decades, yet its mechanism of action is still not certain. There is, however, substantial evidence that lithium exerts neuroprotective effects that are likely downstream from its primary mode of action. Two primary candidates for the direct mechanisms of lithium are the inhibition of glycogen synthase kinase 3β (GSK-3β) and the inhibition of inositol monophosphatase (IMPase). GSK-3β is involved in the regulation of inflammation and is, in general, pro-apoptotic. Specifically, it inhibits transcription factors that would otherwise induce production of cytoprotective proteins such as brain-derived neurotrophic factor (BDNF); thus, its inhibition may be neuroprotective. IMPase indirectly leads to an increase in protein kinase C, which is overactive in mania. Thus, inhibition of IMPase by lithium could potentially reduce manic symptoms.

B Incorrect. Lithium is thought to inhibit GSK-3β and IMPase, not activate them.

C and D Incorrect.

References

Chu CT, Chuang DM. Molecular actions and therapeutic potential of lithium in preclinical and clinical studies of CNS disorders. *Pharmacol Ther* 2010;**128**:281–304.

Pasquali L, Busceti CL, Fulceri F, Paparelli A, Fornai F. Intracellular pathways underlying the effects of lithium. *Behav Pharmacol* 2010;**21**:473–92.

Quiroz JA, Machado-Vieira R, Zarate Jr. CA, Manji HK. Novel insights into lithium's mechanism of action: neurotrophic and neuroprotective effects. *Neuropsychobiology* 2010;**62**:50–60.

QUESTION TWELVE

A 24-year-old man with bipolar disorder is being initiated on lithium, with monitoring of his levels until a therapeutic serum concentration is achieved. Once the patient is stabilized, how often should his serum lithium levels be monitored (excluding one-off situations such as dose or illness change)?

A. Every 2 to 3 months

B. Every 6 to 12 months

C. Every 1 to 2 years

D. Routine monitoring is not necessary

Answer to Question Twelve

The correct answer is B.

Choice	Peer answers
A. Every 2 to 3 months	26%
B. Every 6 to 12 months	74%
C. Every 1 to 2 years	0%
D. Routine monitoring is not necessary	0%

A Incorrect. Initially, lithium levels should be monitored every 1–2 weeks until the desired serum concentration is achieved, and then every 2 to 3 months for the first 6 months. However, this frequency of monitoring is not required once the patient is stabilized.

B Correct. Once a patient is stabilized, lithium levels need only be monitored every 6 to 12 months.

C and D Incorrect.

References

Grandjean EM, Aubry JM. Lithium: updated human knowledge using an evidence-based approach. Part II: Clinical pharmacology and therapeutic monitoring. *CNS Drugs* 2009;**23**(4):331–49.

McKnight RF, Adida M, Budge K, et al. Lithium toxicity profile: a systematic review and meta-analysis. *Lancet* 2012;**379**:721–8.

QUESTION THIRTEEN

A 49-year-old clerk with bipolar disorder has been maintained on 900 mg/day of lithium. She was doing well for a long time and had even been able to lose the weight she had initially gained with lithium. She broke up with her boyfriend 5 months ago and has been feeling depressed ever since. You augment her with 300 mg/day of quetiapine, but after several weeks she complains of weight gain and wants to change medications. Blockade of which two receptors was most likely responsible for this weight gain induced by quetiapine?

A. Serotonin 2A and muscarinic 3

B. Dopamine 2 and alpha 1 adrenergic

C. Muscarinic 1 and serotonin 6

D. Serotonin 2C and histamine 1

Answer to Question Thirteen

The correct answer is D.

Choice	Peer answers
A. Serotonin 2A and muscarinic 3	5%
B. Dopamine 2 and alpha 1 adrenergic	7%
C. Muscarinic 1 and serotonin 6	7%
D. Serotonin 2C and histamine 1	81%

A Incorrect. Blockade of **serotonin 2A** receptors is considered a beneficial property of antipsychotics leading to less extrapyramidal symptoms. Blockade of **muscarinic M3** receptors has been linked to inducing cardiometabolic risk, but has not been linked to weight gain *per se*.

B Incorrect. **Dopamine 2** blockade is the main property of antipsychotics and, if continuous, this blockade can lead to motor side effects, but not to weight gain. **Alpha 1 blockade** can result in decreased blood pressure, dizziness, and drowsiness, but does not lead to weight gain.

C Incorrect. Blockade of **muscarinic M1 receptors** can lead to constipation, blurred vision, dry mouth, and drowsiness, but not weight gain. The function of the **serotonin 6** receptors has not been identified yet.

D Correct. Blockade of **serotonin 2C** receptors and **histamine 1** receptors has been linked to weight gain.

References

Kroeze WK, Hufeisen SJ, Popadak BA, et al. H1-histamine receptor affinity predicts short-term weight gain for typical and atypical antipsychotic drugs. *Neuropsychopharmacology* 2003;**28**(3):519–26.

Schatzberg AF, Nemeroff CB. *Textbook of psychopharmacology*, fourth edition. Washington, DC: American Psychiatric Publishing, Inc.; 2009. (Chapters 28–33)

Stahl SM. *Stahl's essential psychopharmacology*, fourth edition. New York, NY: Cambridge University Press; 2013. (Chapters 5, 8)

Stahl SM, Mignon L. *Stahl's illustrated antipsychotics*, second edition. New York, NY: Cambridge University Press; 2009.

QUESTION FOURTEEN

Ten-year-old Rebecca experienced seizures as a toddler. Her mother took her to a psychiatrist at age 8, because she had violent outbursts of anger, was attacking her older brother, and was severely irritable. That behavior had been going on for the last 6 months. After screening her for ADHD, and other conduct disorders, Dr. Jones had diagnosed her with bipolar I disorder and put her on 800 mg/day of carbamazepine. Over the last few years she has only had a couple of manic episodes but has recently started having frequent debilitating migraines. She has gained weight as well, and now weighs 30 kg (height of 100 cm, BMI=30) and her mother does not want her to start a medication that could lead to more weight gain. Which medication, and at which dose, could be added to her current treatment?

A. 150 mg/day of topiramate (= 5 mg/kg/day)

B. 400 mg/day of topiramate (=13 mg/kg/day)

C. 900 mg/day of lithium

D. 1800 mg/day of lithium

E. 10 mg/day of olanzapine

F. 30 mg/day of olanzapine

Answer to Question Fourteen

The correct answer is A.

Choice	Peer answers
A. 150 mg/day of topiramate (= 5 mg/kg/day)	88%
B. 400 mg/day of topiramate (=13 mg/kg/day)	4%
C. 900 mg/day of lithium	5%
D. 1800 mg/day of lithium	0%
E. 10 mg/day of olanzapine	3%
F. 30 mg/day of olanzapine	0%

A Correct. Besides being used off-label as an adjunct in bipolar disorder, **topiramate** is FDA approved as an anti–migraine medication. It has no weight gain potential, and might even lead to weight loss. Children should be given a lower dose than adults, and the normal dose range for children is 5–9 mg/kg/day.

B Incorrect. This **dose** of topiramate is too high for children.

C and D Incorrect. **Lithium** can be used for vascular headaches, but is not recommended in children, and children tend to have more frequent and severe side effects on lithium. Additionally, lithium can cause weight gain, which is a side effect that the mother wishes to avoid.

E and F Incorrect. The antipsychotic **olanzapine**, while a good adjunct to carbamazepine for breakthrough manic episodes, is highly likely to induce weight gain, and would therefore not be the medication of choice.

References

Schatzberg AF, Nemeroff CB. *Textbook of psychopharmacology*, fourth edition. Washington, DC: American Psychiatric Publishing, Inc.; 2009. (Chapters 62–65)

Stahl SM. *Stahl's essential psychopharmacology*, fourth edition. New York, NY: Cambridge University Press; 2013. (Chapter 8)

Stahl SM. *Stahl's essential psychopharmacology, the prescriber's guide*, fifth edition. New York, NY: Cambridge University Press; 2014.

QUESTION FIFTEEN

A patient with bipolar depression has been treated for 6 months with lamotrigine plus an atypical antipsychotic with partial response. The decision is made to stop the atypical antipsychotic; however, during down-titration, the patient develops withdrawal dyskinesias. No treatment for the dyskinesias is initiated, and after 2 weeks, they still remain. Which of the following is true?

A. If the withdrawal dyskinesias still remain after 2 weeks, they are likely to be permanent

B. Her withdrawal dyskinesias may take several weeks to months to resolve

Answer to Question Fifteen

The correct answer is B.

Choice	Peer answers
A. If the withdrawal dyskinesias still remain after 2 weeks, they are likely to be permanent	8%
B. Her withdrawal dyskinesias may take several weeks to months to resolve	92%

A Incorrect. Withdrawal dyskinesias are often reversible with time and usually resolve within a few weeks; however, they can take several months to resolve, depending on their seriousness. Thus, although the patient's withdrawal dyskinesias still remain after 2 weeks, this does not indicate that they are likely to be permanent.

B Correct. It may take several weeks to months for the patient's withdrawal dyskinesias to resolve.

References

Aia PG, Reveulta GJ, Cloud LJ, Factor SA. Tardive dyskinesia. *Curr Treatment Options Neurol* 2011;**13**(3):231–41.

Moseley CN, Simpson-Khanna HA, Catalano G, Catalano MC. Covert dyskinesia associated with aripiprazole: a case report and review of the literature. *Clin Neuropharmacol* 2013;**36**(4):128–30.

Umbrich P, Soares KV. Benzodiazepines for neuroleptic-induced tardive dyskinesia. *Cochrane Database Syst Rev* 2003;(2):CD000205.

QUESTION SIXTEEN

A patient with bipolar disorder has been taking valproate with only partial control of depressive symptoms, and his clinician elects to add lamotrigine. Compared to lamotrigine monotherapy, what adjustment should be made to the lamotrigine titration schedule in the presence of valproate?

A. Slower titration schedule, same target dose

B. Same titration schedule, half the target dose

C. Slower titration schedule, half the target dose

D. Same titration schedule, same dose

Answer to Question Sixteen

The correct answer is C.

Choice	Peer answers
A. Slower titration schedule, same target dose	5%
B. Same titration schedule, half the target dose	14%
C. Slower titration schedule, half the target dose	78%
D. Same titration schedule, same dose	3%

C Correct. Valproate increases the plasma levels of lamotrigine, so when adding lamotrigine to valproate the target dose is lower and titration is slower (in comparison to initiating lamotrigine monotherapy):

- For the first 2 weeks: 25 mg every other day
- Week 3: increase to 25 mg/day
- Week 5: increase to 50 mg/day
- Week 6: increase to 100 mg/day

A, B, and D Incorrect.

References
Stahl SM. *Essential psychopharmacology, the prescriber's guide*, fifth edition. New York, NY: Cambridge University Press; 2013.

Chapter peer comparison

For the Bipolar disorder and mood stabilizers section, the correct answer was selected 75% of the time.

5 ANXIETY DISORDERS AND ANXIOLYTICS

QUESTION ONE

A 35-year-old female presents to your office and begins to divulge her frequent worries: ever since she was young she was worried someone close to her would die in a freak accident. As she grew older, this worry was exacerbated by the fear that she would pass away without telling her friends and family how important they are to her. Additionally, once she had children, she became so worried for their safety that she rarely lets them leave the house. Furthermore, she has constant worries about how things will work out for her in the future, and recently experienced a panic attack. How might you currently diagnose this patient?

A. Posttraumatic stress disorder

B. Panic disorder

C. Social anxiety disorder

D. Generalized anxiety disorder

Answer to Question One

The correct answer is D.

Choice	Peer answers
A. Posttraumatic stress disorder	1%
B. Panic disorder	1%
C. Social anxiety disorder	1%
D. Generalized anxiety disorder	97%

A   Incorrect. Posttraumatic stress disorder generally originates after a traumatic event; it does not appear that this patient has ever actually experienced a traumatic death experience. She just appears to have excessive worry.

B   Incorrect. Panic disorder is characterized by the presence of spontaneous panic attacks, which this patient does not report having.

C   Incorrect. Worry in social anxiety disorder is tied to embarrassment, whereas this patient's worry is related to a fear of dying.

D   Correct. This patient is displaying core symptoms of generalized anxiety disorder via generalized anxiety and worry. Although she did have a panic attack, a single panic attack is insufficient for a diagnosis of either panic disorder or social anxiety disorder.

References

Schatzberg AF, Nemeroff CB. *Textbook of psychopharmacology*, fourth edition. Washington, DC: American Psychiatric Publishing, Inc.; 2009. (Chapter 47)

Stahl SM. *Stahl's essential psychopharmacology*, fourth edition. New York, NY: Cambridge University Press; 2013. (Chapter 9)

Stahl SM, Grady MM. *Stahl's illustrated anxiety, stress, and PTSD.* New York, NY: Cambridge University Press; 2010. (Chapter 2)

QUESTION TWO

A 35-year-old male Army veteran has been experiencing anxiety attacks during which he has difficulty breathing and increased heart rate. His symptom of difficulty breathing is hypothetically related to activation in the:

A. Hippocampus

B. Hypothalamus

C. Parabrachial nucleus

D. Periaqueductal gray

Answer to Question Two

The correct answer is C.

Choice	Peer answers
A. Hippocampus	19%
B. Hypothalamus	25%
C. Parabrachial nucleus	46%
D. Periaqueductal gray	10%

A Incorrect. The hippocampus is involved in a reciprocal relationship with the amygdala when re-experiencing occurs, a phenomenon often associated with PTSD.

B Incorrect. The hypothalamus regulates endocrine output of fear, which can increase cortisol output, in turn increasing risk of coronary artery disease, type 2 diabetes, and stroke if prolonged activation of hypothalamic pituitary adrenal (HPA) axis is present.

C Correct. The parabrachial nucleus (PBN) regulates changes in respiration, which can occur during fear response. This regulation is activated by the amygdala. Excessive activation of the PBN can lead to an increased rate of respiration and symptoms such as shortness of breath or sense of being smothered.

D Incorrect. The periaqueductal gray is responsible for the fight or flight response often seen during a fear reaction, not the respiratory response.

References

Schatzberg AF, Nemeroff CB. *Textbook of psychopharmacology*, fourth edition. Washington, DC: American Psychiatric Publishing, Inc.; 2009. (Chapters 7, 47)

Stahl SM. *Stahl's essential psychopharmacology*, fourth edition. New York, NY: Cambridge University Press; 2013. (Chapter 9)

Stahl SM, Grady MM. *Stahl's illustrated anxiety, stress, and PTSD*. New York, NY: Cambridge University Press; 2010. (Chapter 1)

QUESTION THREE

A 46-year-old female patient has been experiencing several anxiety-based symptoms for many years, and was previously diagnosed with generalized anxiety disorder. She describes difficulty concentrating in addition to difficulty falling asleep. Her family has recently told her that she seems to be displaying heightened anger responses toward them over minor details. Oftentimes she will cry for extended periods of time and become irritable and distant. Based on the above patient's revelations, if she were to continue to experience these stressful reactions to stimuli (i.e., excessive crying, fatigue, problems concentrating, tension, irritability), what could potentially occur?

A. Increased hippocampal volume

B. Reduced brain-derived neurotrophic factor (BDNF) production

C. Reduced reactivity to stress

D. Decreased hippocampal volume

E. B and D

F. A and C

Answer to Question Three

The correct answer is E.

Choice	Peer answers
A. Increased hippocampal volume	1%
B. Reduced BDNF production	3%
C. Reduced reactivity to stress	1%
D. Decreased hippocampal volume	5%
E. B and D	89%
F. A and C	2%

A and C Incorrect. Hippocampal volume in chronic stress is actually theorized to decrease, not increase. Reduced reactivity to stress may occur in patients who experience mild stressors while growing up, which may result in an improved adaptability when dealing with adult stressors. However, severe or persistent stress, such as this adult is experiencing, does not lead to reduced reactivity to stress.

B and D Correct. Reduced BDNF production can occur in patients who experience chronic stress, leading to a decreased ability to create and maintain neurons and neuronal connections. Decreased hippocampal volume, perhaps related to decreased expression of BDNF, has been reported in some chronic stress conditions such as major depression and certain anxiety disorders. A major treatment strategy for stress-related disorders is the use of selective serotonin reuptake inhibitors (SSRIs), which can increase BDNF levels because serotonin initiates signal transduction cascades that lead to BDNF release.

E Correct; as both B and D are correct answers.

F Incorrect; as both A and C are incorrect answers.

References
Schatzberg AF, Nemeroff CB. *Textbook of psychopharmacology*, fourth edition. Washington, DC: American Psychiatric Publishing, Inc.; 2009. (Chapters 7, 47)

Bremner JD. Stress and brain atrophy. *CNS Neurol Disord Drug Targets* 2006;**5**(5):503–12.

Stahl SM, Grady MM. *Stahl's illustrated anxiety, stress, and PTSD*. New York, NY: Cambridge University Press; 2010. (Chapter 1)

QUESTION FOUR

A 51-year-old male veteran with chronic PTSD has agreed to begin pharmacotherapy for his debilitating symptoms of arousal and anxiety associated with his experiences in Iraq 2 years ago. Which of the following would be appropriate as first-line treatment?

A. Paroxetine

B. Paroxetine or diazepam

C. Paroxetine, diazepam, or D–cycloserine

D. Paroxetine, diazepam, D–cycloserine, or quetiapine

Answer to Question Four

The correct answer is A.

Choice	Peer answers
A. Paroxetine	94%
B. Paroxetine or diazepam	4%
C. Paroxetine, diazepam, or D-cycloserine	2%
D. Paroxetine, diazepam, D-cycloserine, or quetiapine	1%

A Correct. Paroxetine, a selective serotonin-norepinephrine reuptake inhibitor, is approved for use in PTSD.

B Incorrect. Diazepam is a benzodiazepine. Benzodiazepines do not have evidence of efficacy in PTSD and are not generally recommended for first-line use in PTSD.

C Incorrect. D-cycloserine, an NMDA agonist, has been theorized to be useful in facilitating fear extinction, and may be useful in conjunction with exposure therapy. However, it is not a first-line choice.

D Incorrect. Quetiapine, an atypical antipsychotic, is not approved as first-line treatment for PTSD, but may be useful in selected cases as a third-line treatment, specifically for sleep and possible reduction of nightmares.

References

Sauve W, Stahl SM. Psychopharmacological treatment of PTSD. In: *Treating PTSD in military personnel: a clinical handbook.* New York, NY: Guilford Press, 2011.

Schatzberg AF, Nemeroff CB. *Textbook of psychopharmacology,* fourth edition. Washington, DC: American Psychiatric Publishing, Inc.; 2009. (Chapter 56)

Stahl SM, Grady MM. *Stahl's illustrated anxiety, stress, and PTSD.* New York, NY: Cambridge University Press; 2010. (Chapters 4–8)

Stahl SM. *Case studies: Stahl's essential psychopharmacology.* New York, NY: Cambridge University Press; 2011.

Anxiety disorders and anxiolytics

QUESTION FIVE

A 45-year-old female presents with a hand-washing compulsion and an obsession with air fresheners. Based on these symptoms, which of the following is most likely to be true?

A. She may have been born with the catechol-O-methyltransferase (COMT) Met genotype, leading to an increased risk of susceptibility to worry and anxiety disorders.

B. She may have been born with the COMT Val genotype, leading to an increased risk of susceptibility to worry and anxiety disorders.

C. She may have been born with the l variant of the gene for the serotonin transporter (SERT), leading to an increased risk of developing a mood or anxiety disorder.

D. She may have been born with the s variant of the gene for SERT, leading to an increased risk of developing a mood or anxiety disorder.

E. A and D

F. B and C

Answer to Question Five

The correct answer is E.

Choice	Peer answers
A. She may have been born with the catechol-*O*-methyltransferase (COMT) Met genotype, leading to an increased risk of susceptibility to worry and anxiety disorders	9%
B. She may have been born with the COMT Val genotype, leading to an increased risk of susceptibility to worry and anxiety disorders	7%
C. She may have been born with the l variant of the gene for the serotonin transporter (SERT), leading to an increased risk of developing a mood or anxiety disorder	6%
D. She may have been born with the s variant of the gene for SERT, leading to an increased risk of developing a mood or anxiety disorder	7%
E. A and D	51%
F. B and C	21%

A and D Correct. Those born with the COMT Met genotype may be at an increased risk of susceptibility to worry and anxiety disorders. Additionally, those born with the s variant of the gene for SERT appear to be at an increased risk of developing a mood or anxiety disorder.

E Correct, as A and D are correct answers. This patient's OCD may theoretically be linked to either the COMT Met genotype or the s variant of the gene for SERT.

B, C, and F Incorrect. Those born with the COMT Val genotype may be at a reduced risk of developing an anxiety disorder compared to those with the Met genotype. People who carry the l variant of the gene for SERT appear to be more resilient to stress and anxiety than those with the s variant.

References

Lonsdorf TB, Weike AI, Nikamo P, et al. Genetic gating of human fear learning and extinction. *Psychol Sci* 2009;**20**:198–206.

Munafo MR, Brown SM, Hariri AR. Serotonin transporter (5-HTTLPR) genotype and amygdala activation: a meta-analysis. *Biol Psychiatry* 2008;**63**:852–7.

Risch N, Herrel R, Lehner T, et al. Interaction between the serotonin transporter gene (5-HTTLPR), stressful life events, and risk of depression: a meta-analysis. *JAMA* 2009;**301**:2462–71.

Stahl SM, Grady MM. *Stahl's illustrated anxiety, stress, and PTSD.* New York, NY: Cambridge University Press; 2010. (Chapter 1)

QUESTION SIX

A 34-year-old woman with posttraumatic stress disorder has been treated with exposure therapy, with partial success. Her clinician is considering an adjunct medication. The agent D-cycloserine could be efficacious for reducing symptoms in anxiety disorders because it has been shown to:

A. Modulate glutamate neurotransmission during fear conditioning

B. Modulate glutamate neurotransmission during fear extinction

Answer to Question Six

The correct answer is B.

Choice	Peer answers
A. Modulate glutamate neurotransmission during fear conditioning	26%
B. Modulate glutamate neurotransmission during fear extinction	74%

A Incorrect. When an individual encounters a stressful or fearful experience, the sensory input is relayed to the amygdala, where it is integrated with input from the ventromedial prefrontal cortex (VMPFC) and hippocampus, so that a fear response can be either generated or suppressed. The amygdala may "remember" stimuli associated with that experience by increasing the efficiency of glutamate neurotransmission, so that on future exposure to stimuli, a fear response is more efficiently triggered. If this is not countered by input from the VMPFC to suppress the fear response, fear conditioning proceeds. Because D-cycloserine, as an N-methyl-D-aspartate (NMDA) co-agonist, may strengthen the efficiency of glutamate neurotransmission, it would theoretically *increase* rather than decrease the likelihood of fear conditioning.

B Correct. Fear conditioning is not readily reversed, but it can be inhibited through new learning. This new learning is termed fear extinction and is the progressive reduction of the response to a feared stimulus that is repeatedly presented without adverse consequences. Thus the VMPFC and hippocampus learn a new context for the feared stimulus and send input to the amygdala to suppress the fear response. The "memory" of the conditioned fear is still present, however. Strengthening of synapses involved in fear extinction could help enhance the development of fear extinction learning in the amygdala and reduce symptoms of anxiety disorders. Administration of the D-cycloserine while an individual is receiving exposure therapy could increase the efficiency of glutamate neurotransmission at synapses involved in fear extinction.

References
Stahl SM. *Stahl's essential psychopharmacology, the prescriber's guide*, fifth edition. New York, NY: Cambridge University Press; 2014.

Anxiety disorders and anxiolytics

QUESTION SEVEN

A 26-year-old patient with panic disorder is willing to begin pharmacotherapy for treatment of his phobias and panic attacks. Clonazepam is suggested; what would be your recommended dose?

A. 0.25 mg/day to begin, uptitrating to 1 mg/day after 3 days

B. 4 mg/day, uptitrating to 6 mg/day after 1 week

C. 2 mg/day, uptitrating every 3 days until 20 mg/day is reached

D. 1.5 mg/day, uptitrating 0.5 mg/day every other day

Answer to Question Seven

The correct answer is A.

Choice	Peer answers
A. 0.25 mg/day to begin, uptitrating to 1 mg/day after 3 days	87%
B. 4 mg/day, uptitrating to 6 mg/day after 1 week	1%
C. 2 mg/day, uptitrating every 3 days until 20 mg/day is reached	0%
D. 1.5 mg/day, uptitrating 0.5 mg/day every other day	12%

A Correct. For panic disorder, the general recommended dose is 0.25 mg/day divided into two doses, raised to 1 mg after 3 days dosed twice daily or once at bedtime.

B Incorrect. Maximum dose is generally 4 mg/day. 4 mg/day is usually considered the maximum dose for panic disorder, not the starting dose.

C Incorrect. 2 mg/day is not the general recommended starting dose for panic disorder. Additionally, 20 mg/day is the maximum dose for seizures, not panic disorder.

D Incorrect. 1.5 mg/day is generally the starting dose recommended for seizures, not panic disorder.

References

Schatzberg AF, Nemeroff CB. *Textbook of psychopharmacology*, fourth edition. Washington, DC: American Psychiatric Publishing, Inc.; 2009. (Chapter 24)

Stahl SM. *Stahl's essential psychopharmacology, the prescriber's guide*, fifth edition. New York, NY: Cambridge University Press; 2014.

QUESTION EIGHT

A 4-year-old girl has just been removed from her home by social services due to suspicions of abuse and neglect. Severe early life stress can cause changes in functioning of the hypothalamic pituitary adrenal (HPA) axis, which in turn can increase risk for the development of future stress-related disorders. Research suggests that modulation at what level may be necessary in order to prevent the changes in HPA functioning that occur with early stress?

A. Corticotropin releasing hormone (CRH) gene expression/ CRH activity

B. Adrenocorticotropic hormone (ACTH) gene expression/ ACTH activity

C. Cortisol gene expression/cortisol activity

Answer to Question Eight

The correct answer is A.

Choice	Peer answers
A. Corticotropin releasing hormone (CRH) gene expression/CRH activity	62%
B. Adrenocorticotropic hormone (ACTH) gene expression/ACTH activity	10%
C. Cortisol gene expression/cortisol activity	28%

A Correct. Changes in HPA axis functioning that can occur with severe early life stress may begin with the *Crh* gene. That is, changes in *Crh* gene expression precede the other changes that are seen with early mild or severe stress. Thus, in cases of mild stress, it seems that reduced expression of CRH promotes less peptide release in response to stress, and therefore less glucocorticoid release, which ultimately causes upregulation of glucocorticoid receptors. In addition, studies with non-handled rats show that blocking CRH from binding to its type 1 receptor can lead to the same changes and corresponding enhancements in cognitive function. Similarly, blocking CRH1 receptors soon after exposure to early life chronic stress can normalize hippocampal function in adulthood.

The results of these studies suggest that some of the mechanisms behind the risk for stress-related disorders may be set in motion at a very young age. Accordingly, treatment may need to be administered not after symptoms develop, but rather immediately after – or during – exposure to early life stress, in order to prevent the changes in gene expression that may confer greater risk later in life. This may explain why CRH1 antagonists in major depressive disorder in adults – long after possible exposure to early life stressors – have been mostly ineffective.

B, C, and D Incorrect.

References
Korosi A, Baram TZ. Plasticity of the stress response early in life: mechanisms and significance. *Dev Psychobiol* 2010;**52**:661–70.

McClelland S, Korosi A, Cope J, Ivy A, Baram TZ. Emerging roles of epigenetic mechanisms in the enduring effects of early-life stress and experience on learning and memory. *Neurobiol Learning Mem* 2011;**96**(1): 79–88.

QUESTION NINE

A 31-year-old female assault victim is brought to the ER after tracking down passersby for help. She appears rightly traumatized from the incident. Which of the following pharmacotherapy options has been theorized as a potential preemptive treatment to the development of PTSD?

A. *N*-methyl-D-aspartate (NMDA) agonist such as D-cycloserine

B. Alpha 2 delta ligand such as pregabalin

C. Beta adrenergic blocker such as propranolol

D. Benzodiazepine such as diazepam

Answer to Question Nine

The correct answer is C.

Choice	Peer answers
A. N-methyl-D-aspartate (NMDA) agonist such as D-cycloserine	16%
B. Alpha 2 delta ligand such as pregabalin	2%
C. Beta adrenergic blocker such as propranolol	75%
D. Benzodiazepine such as diazepam	7%

A Incorrect. An NMDA agonist is useful in facilitating fear extinction, but would most likely not be helpful in this case, as the trauma has just occurred.

B Incorrect. Alpha 2 delta ligands may be used off-label in the US to treat anxiety, but are often utilized once the disorder has been diagnosed, rather than dealing with an immediate trauma. Preemptive treatment has produced some potentially promising results, if administered within the appropriate window of time from trauma.

C Correct. Beta adrenergic blockers have been shown to block formation of fear conditioning immediately following trauma. Thus, in this case, propranolol may be theoretically useful (off-label) to aid in decreasing risk of developing an anxiety disorder like posttraumatic stress disorder due to her incident.

D Incorrect. Benzodiazepines are commonly used to treat established anxiety disorders, rather than to preempt the development of an anxiety disorder.

References

Orr SP, Milad MR, Metzger LJ, Lasko NB, Gilbertson MW, Pitman RK. Effects of beta blockade, PTSD diagnosis, and explicit threat on the extinction and retention of an aversively conditioned response. *Biol Psychol* 2006;**732**:262–71.

Sauve W, Stahl SM. Psychopharmacological treatment of PTSD. In: *Treating PTSD in military personnel: a clinical handbook*. New York, NY: Guilford Press, 2011.

Schatzberg AF, Nemeroff CB. *Textbook of psychopharmacology*, fourth edition. Washington, DC: American Psychiatric Publishing, Inc.; 2009. (Chapter 56)

Stahl SM, Grady MM. *Stahl's illustrated anxiety, stress, and PTSD*. New York, NY: Cambridge University Press; 2010. (Chapters 4–8)

Stahl SM. *Case studies: Stahl's essential psychopharmacology*. New York, NY: Cambridge University Press; 2011.

Anxiety disorders and anxiolytics

QUESTION TEN

A man who was severely bitten by a dog as a child is beginning cognitive restructuring therapy to treat his posttraumatic stress disorder (PTSD). He identifies walking down the sidewalk past a person with their dog on a leash as a highly distressing situation, rating his fear during such an encounter as 80/100. He states that he strongly believes any dog is likely to escape its leash and attack him. The next step in cognitive restructuring would be for him to:

A. Put himself in a situation in which he encounters a dog on a leash

B. Identify evidence for and against the thought that the dog would escape and attack him

C. Practice techniques such as breathing exercises while thinking about encountering a dog on a leash

Answer to Question Ten

The correct answer is B.

Choice	Peer answers
A. Put himself in a situation in which he encounters a dog on a leash	1%
B. Identify evidence for and against the thought that the dog would escape and attack him	63%
C. Practice techniques such as breathing exercises while thinking about encountering a dog on a leash	36%

A Incorrect. Putting himself in a situation in which he encounters his fear (i.e., a dog) would be part of exposure therapy, but is not part of cognitive restructuring.

B Correct. Cognitive restructuring is a process by which patients learn to evaluate and modify inaccurate and unhelpful thoughts (e.g., "All dogs are vicious"). There are six main steps of cognitive restructuring: (1) identify a distressing event/thought; (2) identify and rate (0–100) emotions related to the event/thought; (3) identify automatic thoughts associated with the emotions, rate the degree to which one believes them, and select one to challenge; (4) identify evidence in support of and against the thought; (5) generate a response to the thought using the evidence for/against (even though <evidence for>, in fact <evidence against>) and rate the degree of belief in the response; and (6) rerate emotion related to the event/thought.

C Incorrect. Breathing exercises are not part of cognitive restructuring.

References
Stahl SM, Grady MM. *Stahl's illustrated anxiety, stress, and PTSD.* New York, NY: Cambridge University Press; 2010. (Chapter 6)

Zayfert C, Becker CB. *Cognitive-behavioral therapy for PTSD: a case formulation approach.* New York, NY: The Guildford Press; 2007.

Anxiety disorders and anxiolytics

QUESTION ELEVEN

A patient presents with comorbid PTSD and substance abuse. Her care provider recommends seeking safety therapy as an initial treatment strategy prior to beginning any other CBT or medication. This means that:

A. PTSD will be addressed first

B. Substance abuse will be addressed first

C. PTSD and substance abuse will be addressed simultaneously

Answer to Question Eleven

The correct answer is C.

Choice	Peer answers
A. PTSD will be addressed first	12%
B. Substance abuse will be addressed first	35%
C. PTSD and substance abuse will be addressed simultaneously	52%

C   Correct. Seeking safety therapy is a technique specifically developed for individuals with substance abuse and trauma histories. It is an integrated treatment approach in which both PTSD and substance abuse are addressed simultaneously, with the main goal being to help patients attain safety in their lives (in terms of relationships, thought processes, behaviors, and emotions).

A and B   Incorrect.

References
Stahl SM, Grady MM. *Stahl's illustrated anxiety, stress, and PTSD.* New York, NY: Cambridge University Press; 2010. (Chapter 6)

Zayfert C, Becker CB. *Cognitive-behavioral therapy for PTSD: a case formulation approach.* New York, NY: The Guildford Press; 2007.

QUESTION TWELVE

A 57-year-old man presents with depression and a history of obsessive compulsive symptoms that began in his twenties and are mostly religious in nature. He has not responded to numerous previous trials of serotonergic medications at typical depression doses. He fairly recently began cognitive behavioral therapy (CBT) and has responded well to it; however, he continues to experience significant symptoms of OCD, rating his symptoms a 7/10 in severity. His current medications include fluoxetine 80 mg/day and trazodone 50 mg/night. Which of the following is true regarding the appropriate dosing of SSRIs in OCD?

A. Doses are typically lower than those in depression

B. Doses are typically the same as those in depression

C. Doses are typically higher than those in depression

Answer to Question Twelve

The correct answer is C.

Choice	Peer answers
A. Doses are typically lower than those in depression	4%
B. Doses are typically the same as those in depression	2%
C. Doses are typically higher than those in depression	94%

A Incorrect (doses are typically lower than those in depression).

B Incorrect (doses are typically the same as those in depression).

C Correct. Higher doses of SSRIs than those used in depression are often needed in OCD, in many cases exceeding the recommended maximum dose:

Recommended daily doses for OCD	
Citalopram	40 mg*
Clomipramine	250 mg
Escitalopram	60 mg
Fluoxetine	120 mg
Fluvoxamine	450 mg
Paroxetine	100 mg
Sertraline	400 mg

* The previous recommended daily dose for citalopram in OCD was 120 mg/day; however, the label for citalopram now includes a warning that it may cause QTc prolongation at doses above 40 mg/day.

References

Abudy A, Juven-Wetzler A, Zohar J. Pharmacological management of treatment-resistant obsessive-compulsive disorder. *CNS Drugs* 2011;**25**(7): 585–96.

QUESTION THIRTEEN

A 38-year-old man with a history of treatment-resistant PTSD has now experienced improvement on quetiapine 300 mg/day, duloxetine 90 mg/day, and zolpidem 10 mg at bedtime. However, he complains of ongoing nightmares and difficulty staying asleep. He was previously initiated on prazosin 3 mg at bedtime, but he experienced intolerable dizziness, and it was discontinued. Can this patient be rechallenged with prazosin? If so, at what dose?

A. Yes; dose should be initiated at 1 mg at bedtime

B. Yes; dose should be initiated at 3 mg at bedtime

C. No; prazosin is contraindicated with quetiapine

D. No; prazosin should not be reattempted in patients with previous intolerability

Answer to Question Thirteen

The correct answer is A.

Choice	Peer answers
A. Yes; dose should be initiated at 1 mg at bedtime	88%
B. Yes; dose should be initiated at 3 mg at bedtime	0%
C. No; prazosin is contraindicated with quetiapine	6%
D. No; prazosin should not be reattempted in patients with previous intolerability	7%

A Correct. Prazosin, an alpha 1 antagonist, can be an effective treatment for nightmares in PTSD. The initial dose of prazosin should be 1 mg at bedtime and titrated up 1 mg every 2–3 days to decrease the risk of syncope.

B Incorrect. There is risk of "first dose effect" syncope with sudden loss of consciousness (1%) with an initial dose of at least 2 mg; thus, 3 mg would be too high for an initiation dose.

C Incorrect. Prazosin is not contraindicated with quetiapine. The only contraindications for prazosin are proven allergy to prazosin or to quinazolines (e.g., the cancer medications gefitinib and erlotinib or the prostatic hyperplasia medications alfuzosin and bunazosin).

D Incorrect. There is no reason why a patient cannot be rechallenged with prazosin if they experienced previous intolerability (assuming they did not have an allergic reaction). Patients may require slower titration or lower dose if they have previously not tolerated prazosin.

References
Kung A, Espinel Z, Lalpid MI. Treatment of nightmares with prazosin: a systematic review. *Mayo Clin Proc* 2012;**87**(9):890–900.

Stahl SM. *Stahl's essential psychopharmacology, the prescriber's guide*, fifth edition. New York, NY: Cambridge University Press; 2014.

Anxiety disorders and anxiolytics

QUESTION FOURTEEN

A 28-year-old combat veteran with PTSD has not responded to multiple trials of oral medication. He suffers from nightmares, rarely maintains sleep longer than 2 hours, and has lost interest in his family life, which is particularly difficult for his wife given that she is pregnant with their first child. The role of glutamate in traumatic memory formation and extinction suggests that ketamine may be beneficial; however, the potential side-effect profile of ketamine could also be concerning for patients with PTSD. In a recent controlled proof-of-concept study in PTSD, ketamine:

A. Did not reduce PTSD symptoms and caused transient worsening of dissociative symptoms

B. Did not reduce PTSD symptoms and caused sustained worsening of dissociative symptoms

C. Reduced PTSD symptoms and caused transient worsening of dissociative symptoms

D. Reduced PTSD symptoms and caused sustained worsening of dissociative symptoms

Answer to Question Fourteen

The correct answer is C.

Choice	Peer answers
A. Did not reduce PTSD symptoms and caused transient worsening of dissociative symptoms	13%
B. Did not reduce PTSD symptoms and caused sustained worsening of dissociative symptoms	3%
C. Reduced PTSD symptoms and caused transient worsening of dissociative symptoms	78%
D. Reduced PTSD symptoms and caused sustained worsening of dissociative symptoms	6%

Like D-cycloserine, ketamine could theoretically strengthen the efficiency of glutamate neurotransmission at synapses involved in fear extinction and thus improve symptoms of PTSD. In a proof-of-concept, double-blind, randomized, crossover trial comparing ketamine to the active placebo control midazolam, researchers found that ketamine infusion was associated with significant reduction in PTSD symptom severity, assessed 24 hours after infusion. This remained significant after adjusting for depressive symptom severity. In the study, ketamine caused transient worsening of dissociative symptoms, but this was not sustained. The clinical relevance of this study will be subject both to successful replication and to identification of an alternate method of ketamine administration. Methods that are under investigation for depression include intranasal and intramuscular.

A Incorrect. It is true that ketamine caused transient worsening of dissociative symptoms; however, it also reduced PTSD symptoms.

B Incorrect. Ketamine caused transient but not sustained worsening of dissociative symptoms.

C Correct. Ketamine reduced PTSD symptoms and caused transient worsening of dissociative symptoms.

D Incorrect (reduced PTSD symptoms and caused sustained worsening of dissociative symptoms).

References

Feder A, Parides MK, Murrough JW, et al. Efficacy of intravenous ketamine for treatment of chronic posttraumatic stress disorder: a randomized clinical trial. *JAMA Psychiatry* 2014;**71**(6):681–8.

Anxiety disorders and anxiolytics

Womble AL. Effects of ketamine on major depressive disorder in a patient with posttraumatic stress disorder. *AANA J* 2013;**81**(2):118–9.

Chapter peer comparison

For the Anxiety disorders and anxiolytics section, the correct answer was selected 75% of the time.

6 CHRONIC PAIN AND ITS TREATMENT

QUESTION ONE

A 34-year-old woman with fibromyalgia, generalized anxiety disorder, and depression is currently taking several psychotropic medications, including alprazolam, duloxetine, hydrocodone/acetaminophen, and pregabalin. She continues to have residual pain, anxiety, and mood symptoms. Her clinician is considering simplifying her medication regimen and plans to discontinue the medication with the least evidence of efficacy for her disorders. Which of the following should be discontinued?

A. Alprazolam

B. Duloxetine

C. Hydrocodone/acetaminophen

D. Pregabalin

Answer to Question One

The correct answer is C.

Choice	Peer answers
A. Alprazolam	24%
B. Duloxetine	0%
C. Hydrocodone/acetaminophen	71%
D. Pregabalin	5%

A Incorrect. Alprazolam is an effective treatment for generalized anxiety disorder.

B Incorrect. Duloxetine is an effective treatment for both depression and for fibromyalgia.

C Correct. Hydrocodone/acetaminophen does not have evidence of efficacy for the treatment of fibromyalgia, nor is it an appropriate treatment for her other illnesses.

D Incorrect. Pregabalin is an effective treatment for fibromyalgia and also has evidence of efficacy in anxiety.

References

Ballantyne JC, Shin NS. Efficacy of opioids for chronic pain: a review of the evidence. *Clin J Pain* 2008;**24**:469–78.

Clauw DJ. Fibromyalgia: an overview. *Am J Med* 2009;**122**(Suppl 12):S3–13.

QUESTION TWO

A 35-year-old woman complains of widespread pain so debilitating that she has been unable to work for the last several weeks, though she did not experience any significant injury that seems to account for the pain. Specifically, she states that even the mild pressure of being touched causes such significant pain that she cringes when her 2-year-old daughter tries to hug her. This type of pain is called:

A. Acute pain

B. Allodynia

C. Hyperalgesia

D. Neuropathic pain

Chronic pain and its treatment

Answer to Question Two

The correct answer is B.

Choice	Peer answers
A. Acute pain	2%
B. Allodynia	49%
C. Hyperalgesia	44%
D. Neuropathic pain	5%

A Incorrect. Acute pain refers to pain that resolves after a short duration and that is usually directly related to the healing of tissue damage. In this case the patient has had significant pain for several weeks despite the lack of any apparent injury; thus, this does not appear to be acute pain.

B Correct. Allodynia is a painful response to a stimulus that does not normally provoke pain, such as pain in response to light touch. This is consistent with what the patient describes.

C Incorrect. Hyperalgesia is an exaggerated pain response to something that is normally painful (for example, extreme pain in response to a pin prick). Mild pressure from being hugged by one's child would not normally elicit pain, and thus this particular complaint does not represent hyperalgesia.

D Incorrect. Neuropathic pain is pain that arises from damage to or dysfunction of any part of the peripheral or central nervous system. Neuropathic pain is not defined by the degree of pain in response to a certain type of stimulus, which is what this patient is describing.

References
McMahon S, Koltzenburg M (eds). *Wall and Melzack's textbook of pain*, fifth edition. London: Harcourt Publishers; 2005.

Stahl SM. *Stahl's essential psychopharmacology*, fourth edition. New York, NY: Cambridge University Press; 2013. (Chapter 10)

Stahl SM. *Stahl's illustrated chronic pain and fibromyalgia*. New York, NY: Cambridge University Press; 2009. (Chapters 3–4)

Chronic pain and its treatment

QUESTION THREE

A young man arrives at the emergency room in great pain after receiving a chemical burn during an accident at work. Which primary afferent neurons would have responded to the chemical stimulus to produce nociceptive neuronal activity?

A. A beta fiber neurons

B. A delta fiber neurons

C. C fiber neurons

Answer to Question Three

The correct answer is C.

Choice	Peer answers
A. A beta fiber neurons	10%
B. A delta fiber neurons	35%
C. C fiber neurons	55%

A   Incorrect. A beta fibers respond to non-noxious small movements such as light touch, hair movement, and vibrations, and do not respond to noxious stimuli.

B   Incorrect. A delta fibers fall somewhere in between A beta fibers and C fiber neurons, sensing noxious mechanical stimuli and subnoxious thermal stimuli.

C   Correct. C fiber peripheral terminals are bare nerve endings that are only activated by noxious mechanical, thermal, or chemical stimuli. Thus C fiber neurons are the primary afferent neurons responsible for nociceptive conduction following this patient's injury.

References

McMahon S, Koltzenburg M (eds). *Wall and Melzack's textbook of pain*, fifth edition. London: Harcourt Publishers; 2005.

Stahl SM. *Stahl's essential psychopharmacology*, fourth edition. New York, NY: Cambridge University Press; 2013. (Chapter 10)

Stahl SM. *Stahl's illustrated chronic pain and fibromyalgia*. New York, NY: Cambridge University Press; 2009. (Chapter 2)

QUESTION FOUR

A 29-year-old woman has just been diagnosed with major depressive disorder and is being prescribed a selective serotonin reuptake inhibitor (SSRI). In addition to depressed mood, lack of interest in her work or friends, and difficulty sleeping, she has been experiencing aches and pains in her arms, shoulders, and torso. She asks if the SSRI is likely to alleviate her painful physical symptoms as well as her emotional ones. Which of the following statements is true?

A. SSRIs may have inconsistent effects on pain because serotonin can both inhibit and facilitate ascending nociceptive signals

B. SSRIs may worsen pain because serotonin can facilitate but not inhibit ascending nociceptive signals

C. SSRIs generally alleviate pain because serotonin can inhibit but not facilitate ascending nociceptive signals

D. SSRIs generally have no effect on pain because serotonin neither facilitates nor inhibits nociceptive signals

Answer to Question Four

The correct answer is A.

Choice	Peer answers
A. SSRIs may have inconsistent effects on pain because serotonin can both inhibit and facilitate ascending nociceptive signals	53%
B. SSRIs may worsen pain because serotonin can facilitate but not inhibit ascending nociceptive signals	0%
C. SSRIs generally alleviate pain because serotonin can inhibit but not facilitate ascending nociceptive signals	26%
D. SSRIs generally have no effect on pain because serotonin neither facilitates nor inhibits nociceptive signals	21%

Two important descending pathways that inhibit ascending nociceptive signals are the noradrenergic and the serotonergic pathways. Thus enhancement of neurotransmission in either of these pathways could contribute to alleviation of chronic pain.

However, serotonin is also a major neurotransmitter in descending facilitation pathways to the spinal cord. The combination of both inhibitory and facilitatory actions of serotonin may explain why SSRIs seem to have inconsistent effects on painful somatic symptoms.

A Correct.

B, C, and D Incorrect.

References

Schatzberg AF, Nemeroff CB. *Textbook of psychopharmacology*, fourth edition. Washington, DC: American Psychiatric Publishing, Inc.; 2009. (Chapters 28, 66)

Stahl SM. *Stahl's essential psychopharmacology*, fourth edition. New York, NY: Cambridge University Press; 2013. (Chapter 10)

Stahl SM. *Stahl's illustrated chronic pain and fibromyalgia*. New York, NY: Cambridge University Press; 2009. (Chapter 5)

QUESTION FIVE

A 22-year-old woman with pain throughout her body, extreme fatigue, and poor sleep is diagnosed with fibromyalgia. Her care provider considers prescribing pregabalin, which may alleviate pain by:

A. Binding to the closed conformation of voltage-sensitive sodium channels

B. Binding to the open conformation of voltage-sensitive sodium channels

C. Binding to the closed conformation of voltage-sensitive calcium channels

D. Binding to the open conformation of voltage-sensitive calcium channels

Chronic pain and its treatment

Answer to Question Five

The correct answer is D.

Choice	Peer answers
A. Binding to the closed conformation of voltage-sensitive sodium channels	7%
B. Binding to the open conformation of voltage-sensitive sodium channels	25%
C. Binding to the closed conformation of voltage-sensitive calcium channels	19%
D. Binding to the open conformation of voltage-sensitive calcium channels	49%

A and B Incorrect. Both voltage-sensitive sodium and voltage-sensitive calcium channels are involved in transmission of pain; however, pregabalin does not bind to voltage-sensitive sodium channels in any conformation.

D Correct. Pregabalin does, however, bind to the alpha 2 delta subunit of voltage-sensitive calcium channels (VSCCs). In fact, pregabalin binds preferentially to the open conformation of these channels and thus may be particularly effective in blocking channels that are the most active, with a "use-dependent" form of inhibition.

C Incorrect. This molecular action predicts more affinity for VSCCs that are actively conducting neuronal impulses within the pain pathway and thus a selective action on those VSCCs causing neuropathic pain, ignoring other VSCCs that are closed, and thus not interfering with normal neurotransmission in central neurons uninvolved in mediating the pathological pain state.

References

Dooley DJ, Taylor CP, Donevan S, Feltner D. Ca2+ channel alpha 2 delta ligands: novel modulators of neurotransmission. *Trends Pharmacol Sci* 2007;**28**:75–2.

Schatzberg AF, Nemeroff CB. *Textbook of psychopharmacology*, fourth edition. Washington, DC: American Psychiatric Publishing, Inc.; 2009. (Chapters 28, 66)

Stahl SM. *Stahl's essential psychopharmacology*, fourth edition. New York, NY: Cambridge University Press; 2013. (Chapter 10)

Stahl SM. *Stahl's illustrated chronic pain and fibromyalgia*. New York, NY: Cambridge University Press; 2009. (Chapter 5)

Chronic pain and its treatment

QUESTION SIX

A 30-year-old man with juvenile-onset diabetes has begun experiencing throbbing pain, particularly at night. In addition, he states that his body generally feels sensitive all over, so that even the brush of his clothes against his skin can be uncomfortable. These symptoms, indicative of diabetic peripheral neuropathy, may be caused by:

A. Inflammation or damage in the periphery without disturbance in central pain processing

B. Central disturbance in pain processing without damage in the periphery

C. Inflammation or damage in the periphery combined with central disturbance in pain processing

Chronic pain and its treatment

Answer to Question Six

The correct answer is C.

Choice	Peer answers
A. Inflammation or damage in the periphery without disturbance in central pain processing	28%
B. Central disturbance in pain processing without damage in the periphery	5%
C. Inflammation or damage in the periphery combined with central disturbance in pain processing	67%

A and B Incorrect.

C Correct. Chronic pain syndromes may be peripheral, central, or both peripheral and central ("mixed") in origin. Over time, diabetes can cause inflammation that damages peripheral nerves and thus leads to painful physical symptoms. In addition, that damage may cause repetitive activation of nociception, and such ongoing neuronal activity may induce central plasticity within the pain pathway, with progressive and potentially irreversible molecular changes in pain processing pathways eventually leading to progressive and potentially irreversible pain symptoms. Thus diabetic peripheral neuropathy is a syndrome in which definite peripheral injury is combined with central sensitization.

References

Stahl SM. *Stahl's essential psychopharmacology*, fourth edition. New York, NY: Cambridge University Press; 2013. (Chapter 10)

Stahl SM. *Stahl's illustrated chronic pain and fibromyalgia*. New York, NY: Cambridge University Press; 2009. (Chapter 2)

QUESTION SEVEN

A 36-year-old woman has just been diagnosed with fibromyalgia. In addition to her painful physical symptoms, she is experiencing problems with memory and significant difficulty concentrating at work. Which of the following may be most likely to alleviate both her physical pain and her cognitive symptoms?

A. Bupropion

B. Cyclobenzaprine

C. Milnacipran

D. Pregabalin

Answer to Question Seven

The correct answer is C.

Choice	Peer answers
A. Bupropion	23%
B. Cyclobenzaprine	4%
C. Milnacipran	51%
D. Pregabalin	23%

Documented mechanisms for alleviating central neuropathic pain include enhancement of serotonergic and noradrenergic neurotransmission in descending spinal pathways as well as reduction of calcium influx in pain pathways. Cognitive dysfunction may be alleviated by increasing dopaminergic (and possibly noradrenergic) neurotransmission in the dorsolateral prefrontal cortex.

A Incorrect. Bupropion is a norepinephrine and dopamine reuptake inhibitor (NDRI) and may reduce cognitive symptoms associated with fibromyalgia when used as adjunct, but is not documented to reduce pain.

B Incorrect. Cyclobenzaprine is a muscle relaxant and may be used for fibromyalgia, but is not generally a first-line choice and does not have efficacy for cognitive symptoms.

C Correct. Milnacipran is a serotonin-norepinephrine reuptake inhibitor (SNRI) with documented efficacy for treating neuropathic pain. In addition, it can also improve cognitive symptoms through its potent norepinephrine reuptake binding property.

D Incorrect. Pregabalin binds to the alpha 2 delta subunit of voltage-sensitive calcium channels to reduce calcium influx. It has documented efficacy for treating neuropathic pain, but is not documented to reduce cognitive symptoms.

References

Schatzberg AF, Nemeroff CB. *Textbook of psychopharmacology*, fourth edition. Washington, DC: American Psychiatric Publishing, Inc.; 2009. (Chapter 66)

Stahl SM. *Stahl's essential psychopharmacology*, fourth edition. New York, NY: Cambridge University Press; 2013. (Chapter 10)

Stahl SM. *Case studies: Stahl's essential psychopharmacology*. New York, NY: Cambridge University Press; 2011.

QUESTION EIGHT

A 60-year-old woman was diagnosed with fibromyalgia 1 year ago but has not responded well to pregabalin, gabapentin, or duloxetine. She is hesitant to take multiple medications and instead hopes to try a different monotherapy. Of the following options, which is the best choice as a second-line monotherapy for fibromyalgia?

A. Amitriptyline

B. Atomoxetine

C. Ibuprofen

D. Modafinil

Answer to Question Eight

The correct answer is A.

Choice	Peer answers
A. Amitriptyline	88%
B. Atomoxetine	7%
C. Ibuprofen	2%
D. Modafinil	4%

A Correct. Amitriptyline is a tricyclic antidepressant that inhibits both the serotonin and norepinephrine transporters. Although it is not generally used first-line for fibromyalgia, it does have documented efficacy in this disorder and is a good second-line option.

B Incorrect. Atomoxetine is a selective norepinephrine reuptake inhibitor (NRI) and may be used as an adjunct for fibromyalgia, particularly for resolution of cognitive symptoms, but does not have documented efficacy for pain and would not be a good choice as a monotherapy.

C Incorrect. Ibuprofen is a nonsteroidal anti-inflammatory agent (NSAID) and can be used to treat pain related to peripheral injury, but it does not have any documented efficacy for fibromyalgia.

D Incorrect. Modafinil is a wake-promoting agent that seems to affect the histaminergic and dopaminergic neurotransmitter systems. It may be a useful adjunct for fatigue in fibromyalgia but does not have documented efficacy for pain.

References

Schatzberg AF, Nemeroff CB. *Textbook of psychopharmacology*, fourth edition. Washington, DC: American Psychiatric Publishing, Inc.; 2009. (Chapter 66)

Stahl SM. *Stahl's essential psychopharmacology*, fourth edition. New York, NY: Cambridge University Press; 2013. (Chapter 10)

Stahl SM. *Stahl's essential psychopharmacology, the prescriber's guide*, fifth edition. New York, NY: Cambridge University Press; 2014.

QUESTION NINE

A 44-year-old male patient with chronic hepatitis is seeking treatment for chronic neuropathic pain. Which of the following would you most likely avoid prescribing for this patient?

A. Duloxetine

B. Gabapentin

C. Pregabalin

Answer to Question Nine

The correct answer is A.

Choice	Peer answers
A. Duloxetine	67%
B. Gabapentin	23%
C. Pregabalin	10%

All of these medications can be effective for chronic neuropathic pain; what distinguishes them here is their effects in hepatic impairment.

A Correct. Duloxetine increases the risk of elevation of serum transaminase levels and is not recommended for use in individuals with hepatic insufficiency; thus it would not be recommended in this case.

B and C Incorrect. Gabapentin and pregabalin are not metabolized by the liver, nor do they appear to have effects on liver functioning; thus they are considered safe in hepatic impairment and do not generally require dose adjustment.

References

Scholz BA, Hammonds CL, Boomershine CS. Duloxetine for the management of fibromyalgia syndrome. *J Pain Res* 2009;**2**:99–108.

Stahl SM. *Stahl's essential psychopharmacology, the prescriber's guide*, fifth edition. New York, NY: Cambridge University Press; 2014.

QUESTION TEN

A 28-year-old patient with a long history of painful somatic symptoms has been diagnosed with major depressive disorder but has not responded to multiple successive trials of selective serotonin reuptake inhibitors (SSRIs). Her clinician is now considering prescribing a monoamine oxidase inhibitor (MAOI). Due to her history of chronic pain, she is currently taking an opioid. Which of the following opioids would be of greatest concern for this patient?

A. Codeine

B. Morphine

C. Hydrocodone

D. Meperidine

Answer to Question Ten

The correct answer is D.

Choice	Peer answers
A. Codeine	4%
B. Morphine	16%
C. Hydrocodone	11%
D. Meperidine	70%

There is no interaction of MAOIs with opioid mechanisms; however, some opioids have serotonergic properties that could increase risk of serotonin syndrome if they were administered together.

A Incorrect. Codeine does not have serotonergic properties and is safe to prescribe with SSRIs.

B Incorrect. Morphine does not have serotonergic properties and is safe to prescribe with SSRIs.

C Incorrect. Hydrocodone does not have serotonergic properties and is safe to prescribe with SSRIs.

D Correct. Meperidine is a potent serotonin reuptake inhibitor and should not be prescribed with MAOIs.

References

Wimbiscus M, Kostenko O, Malone D. MAO inhibitors: risks, benefits, and lore. *Curr Drug Therapy* 2010;**77**(2):859–82.

Stahl SM, Felker A. Monoamine oxidase inhibitors: a modern guide to an unrequited class of antidepressants.*CNS Spectr* 2008;**13**(10):855–70.

Chapter peer comparison

For the Chronic pain and its treatment section, the correct answer was selected 52% of the time.

7 DISORDERS OF SLEEP AND WAKEFULNESS AND THEIR TREATMENT

QUESTION ONE

Denise is a 32-year-old patient with shift work disorder who reports that she is having difficulty in her job as a pastry chef due to excessive sleepiness during her shift. Which of the following is a potential therapeutic mechanism to promote wakefulness?

A. Inhibit GABA activity

B. Inhibit histamine activity

C. Inhibit orexin activity

D. All of the above

E. None of the above

Answer to Question One

The correct answer is A.

Choice	Peer answers
A. Inhibit GABA activity	43%
B. Inhibit histamine activity	4%
C. Inhibit orexin activity	7%
D. All of the above	37%
E. None of the above	9%

The hypothalamus is a key control center for sleep and wake, and the specific circuitry that regulates sleep/wake is called the sleep/wake switch. The "off" setting, or sleep promoter, is localized within the ventrolateral preoptic nucleus (VLPO) of the hypothalamus, while "on" – the wake promoter – is localized within the tuberomammillary nucleus (TMN) of the hypothalamus. Two key neurotransmitters regulate the sleep/wake switch: histamine from the TMN and GABA from the VLPO.

A Correct. When the VLPO is active and GABA is released to the TMN, the sleep promoter is on and the wake promoter is inhibited. Thus, inhibiting GABA activity can promote wakefulness.

B Incorrect. When the TMN is active and histamine is released to the cortex and the VLPO, the wake promoter is on and the sleep promoter is inhibited. Thus, inhibiting histamine activity can promote sleep, not wakefulness.

C Incorrect. The sleep/wake switch is also regulated by orexin neurons in the lateral hypothalamus, which stabilize wakefulness. Inhibition of orexin would therefore promote sleep, not wakefulness. In fact, a deficiency of orexin is an underlying cause of the extreme and sudden sleepiness seen in narcolepsy.

D and E Incorrect.

References
Stahl SM. *Stahl's essential psychopharmacology*, fourth edition. New York, NY: Cambridge University Press; 2013. (Chapter 11)

QUESTION TWO

A 42-year-old police officer presents with sleep cycle disturbances. After sufficient consultation you prescribe her eszopiclone. Which receptors are primarily being targeted by this treatment?

A. Histamine 1

B. Histamine 2

C. Serotonin 2C

D. GABA$_A$ alpha 1 isoform

E. GABA$_A$ alpha 2 and 3 isoforms

Answer to Question Two

The correct answer is D.

Choice	Peer answers
A. Histamine 1	4%
B. Histamine 2	8%
C. Serotonin 2C	4%
D. GABA$_A$ alpha 1 isoform	58%
E. GABA$_A$ alpha 2 and 3 isoforms	27%

A and B Incorrect. Histamine 1, histamine 2, and histamine 3 are targets of both sleep- and wake-promoting agents including histamine releasers, antihistamines, and selective histamine antagonists.

C Incorrect. Serotonin 2C antagonism can be sedating and is one of the targets of some sleep agents, including trazodone and agomelatine.

D Correct. Eszopiclone is a positive allosteric modulator at GABA$_A$ receptors. Eszopiclone primarily targets receptors containing the alpha 1 isoform and this is responsible for its effects on sleep.

E Incorrect. Although eszopiclone may target GABA A receptors that contain the alpha 2 and 3 isoforms, this is not its primary action nor is it related to the sleep effects. Instead, alpha 2 and 3 receptor subtypes are related to anxiolytic, muscle relaxant, and alcohol-potentiating factors.

References
Monti JM, Pandi-Perumal SR. Eszopiclone: its use in the treatment of insomnia. *Neuropsychiatr Dis Treat* 2007;**3**(4):441–53.

Schatzberg AF, Nemeroff CB. *Textbook of psychopharmacology*, fourth edition. Washington, DC: American Psychiatric Publishing, Inc.; 2009. (Chapter 42)

Stahl SM. *Stahl's essential psychopharmacology*, fourth edition. New York, NY: Cambridge University Press; 2013. (Chapter 11)

QUESTION THREE

A 72-year-old woman has been having difficulty sleeping for several weeks, including both difficulty falling asleep and frequent nighttime awakenings. Medical examination rules out an underlying condition contributing to insomnia, and she is not taking any medications that are associated with disrupted sleep. The patient is retired and spends the day caring for her grandchildren, including driving the older ones to school in the morning. Which of the following would be the most appropriate treatment option for this patient?

A. Flurazepam

B. Temazepam

C. Zaleplon

D. Zolpidem CR

Answer to Question Three

The correct answer is D.

Choice	Peer answers
A. Flurazepam	0%
B. Temazepam	6%
C. Zaleplon	30%
D. Zolpidem CR	64%

The half-lives of hypnotics can have an important impact on their tolerability and efficacy profiles.

A Incorrect. Hypnotics with ultra-long half-lives (greater than 24 hours: for example, flurazepam and quazepam) can cause drug accumulation with chronic use. This can cause impairment that has been associated with increased risk of falls, particularly in the elderly.

B Incorrect. Hypnotics with moderate half-lives (15–30 hours: estazolam, temazepam, most tricyclic antidepressants, mirtazapine, olanzapine) may not wear off until after the individual needs to awaken and thus may have "hangover" effects (sedation, memory problems). Given that the patient needs to drive early in the morning, this may not be the best option for her.

C Incorrect. Hypnotics with ultra-short half-lives (1–3 hours: zaleplon, triazolam, zolpidem, melatonin, ramelteon) can wear off before the individual needs to awaken and thus cause loss of sleep maintenance, which is already a problem for this patient.

D Correct. Hypnotics with half-lives that are short but not ultra-short (approximately 6 hours: zolpidem CR, eszopiclone, and perhaps low doses of trazodone or doxepin) may provide rapid onset of action and plasma levels above the minimally effective concentration only for the duration of a normal night's sleep. Thus, of the answer choices, zolpidem CR may best treat the patient's difficulties with sleep onset and maintenance while avoiding risks associated with agents with longer half-lives. The dose of zolpidem CR in eldery patients is 6.25 mg/night.

References

Schatzberg AF, Nemeroff CB. *Textbook of psychopharmacology*, fourth edition. Washington, DC: American Psychiatric Publishing, Inc.; 2009. (Chapter 42)

Stahl SM. *Stahl's essential psychopharmacology*, fourth edition. New York, NY: Cambridge University Press; 2013. (Chapter 11)

Stahl SM. *Stahl's essential psychopharmacology, the prescriber's guide*, fifth edition. New York, NY: Cambridge University Press; 2014.

Disorders of sleep and wakefulness and their treatment

QUESTION FOUR

A 33-year-old man taking estazolam to help him sleep through the night complains that his symptoms have returned despite his adherence to the medication regimen for the past 6 months. You suspect he has developed a tolerance to this drug and elect to switch him to:

A. Temazepam

B. Ramelteon

C. Trazodone

D. Chlordiazepoxide

Answer to Question Four

The correct answer is C.

Choice	Peer answers
A. Temazepam	0%
B. Ramelteon	16%
C. Trazodone	82%
D. Chlordiazepoxide	2%

With long-term use, benzodiazepine hypnotics can cause tolerance and, if discontinued, withdrawal effects.

A and D Incorrect. Because this patient has developed tolerance to his current benzodiazepine, another benzodiazepine such as temazepam and chlordiazepoxide may not be the best choices.

B Incorrect. Ramelteon has not been reported to cause tolerance and can be used for sleep initiation; however, it is not necessarily used for sleep maintenance.

C Correct. Trazodone works by a serotonergic and histaminergic mechanism unique from estazolam and may be able both to induce sleep and suppress any mild withdrawal insomnia when estazolam is stopped. However, if severe insomnia results from estazolam discontinuation, a tapering of this may be necessary until rebound insomnia resolves, while adding trazodone.

References

Carson S, McDonagh MS, Thakurta S, Yen PY. Drug class review: newer drugs for insomnia: final report update 2 [Internet]. *Drug Class Reviews*; 2008.

Schatzberg AF, Nemeroff CB. *Textbook of psychopharmacology*, fourth edition. Washington, DC: American Psychiatric Publishing, Inc.; 2009. (Chapter 60)

Stahl SM. *Stahl's essential psychopharmacology*, third edition. New York, NY: Cambridge University Press; 2008. (Chapter 16)

Stahl SM. *Case studies: Stahl's essential psychopharmacology*. New York, NY: Cambridge University Press; 2011.

QUESTION FIVE

A 75-year-old man in good physical shape is having sleep problems. He wakes up at 4 am and although he tries to stay awake in the evening to prevent this early rising, he usually falls asleep right after dinner, often before 7 pm. Which of the following treatment options may be most beneficial for this patient?

A. Early morning melatonin

B. Evening melatonin

C. Late afternoon/evening light

D. A and C

E. A and B

F. B and C

Answer to Question Five

The correct answer is D.

Choice	Peer answers
A. Early morning melatonin	6%
B. Evening melatonin	8%
C. Late afternoon/evening light	8%
D. A and C	47%
E. A and B	0%
F. B and C	31%

A and C Partially correct.

B, E, and F Incorrect. Evening melatonin would not be appropriate for this patient who is phase-advanced. Rather, evening melatonin (and morning light) may benefit patients with phase-delayed circadian rhythms, potentially resetting the suprachiasmatic nucleus (SCN) so that the sleep/wake switch turns on earlier.

D Correct. This patient is phase-advanced. Phase-advanced circadian rhythms may benefit from early morning melatonin and evening light, which could help reset the SCN so that the sleep/wake switch stays off longer.

References

Edwards BA, O'Driscoll DM, Ali A, Jordon AS, Trinder J, Malhotra A. Aging and sleep: physiology and pathophysiology. *Semin Respir Crit Care Med* 2010;**31**(5):618–33.

Dodson ER, Zee PC. Therapeutics for circadian rhythm sleep disorders. *Sleep Med Clin* 2010;**5**(4):701–15.

Schatzberg AF, Nemeroff CB. *Textbook of psychopharmacology*, fourth edition. Washington, DC: American Psychiatric Publishing, Inc.; 2009. (Chapter 60)

Stahl SM. *Case studies: Stahl's essential psychopharmacology.* New York, NY: Cambridge University Press; 2011.

Disorders of sleep and wakefulness and their treatment

QUESTION SIX

A 45-year-old woman was prescribed doxepin 10 mg/night for insomnia. She reports that it helped only a little, so she has been increasing the dose, up to 100 mg/night, as an attempt to increase the hypnotic effects (with some success). She also reports dizzy spells and constipation. Which property does doxepin exhibit in higher doses that could be the cause of these side effects?

A. Inhibiting reuptake of serotonin and norepinephrine

B. 5HT2A and 5HT2C antagonism

C. Alpha 1 adrenergic and muscarinic 1 antagonism

D. 5HT2A and 5HT2B antagonism

Answer to Question Six

The correct answer is C.

Choice	Peer answers
A. Inhibiting reuptake of serotonin and norepinephrine	2%
B. 5HT2A and 5HT2C antagonism	2%
C. Alpha 1 adrenergic and muscarinic 1 antagonism	94%
D. 5HT2A and 5HT2B antagonism	2%

A, B and D Incorrect. Higher doses of doxepin inhibit reuptake of serotonin and norepinephrine, but such effects are not likely to explain these side effects.

C Correct. Low-dose doxepin is selective for histamine 1 receptors, which is why it can act as a hypnotic. It is likely that alpha 1 adrenergic and muscarinic 1 receptor antagonism seen with higher doses of doxepin would explain these side effects.

References

Schatzberg AF, Nemeroff CB. *Textbook of psychopharmacology*, fourth edition. Washington, DC: American Psychiatric Publishing, Inc.; 2009. (Chapter 42)

Stahl SM. *Stahl's essential psychopharmacology*, fourth edition. New York, NY: Cambridge University Press; 2013. (Chapter 11)

Stahl SM. *Stahl's essential psychopharmacology, the prescriber's guide*, fifth edition. New York, NY: Cambridge University Press; 2014.

Stahl SM. Selective histamine H1 antagonism: novel hypnotic and pharmacologic actions challenge classical notions of antihistamines. *CNS Spectr* 2008;**13**(12):1027–38.

Disorders of sleep and wakefulness and their treatment

QUESTION SEVEN

Although he sleeps soundly through the night, a 54–year–old man, whom you have previously treated for depression, describes feeling physically exhausted, sometimes with sore muscles, when he wakes up in the morning. His wife reports that she frequently wakes in the middle of the night from his movements. Which of the following tests would you refer him to take?

A. Polysomnograph

B. Multiple sleep latency test

C. Maintenance of wakefulness test

D. A and B

E. B and C

F. A and C

G. A, B, and C

Answer to Question Seven

The correct answer is A.

Choice	Peer answers
A. Polysomnograph	67%
B. Multiple sleep latency test	4%
C. Maintenance of wakefulness test	2%
D. A and B	13%
E. B and C	2%
F. A and C	4%
G. A, B, and C	8%

A Correct. It is likely that this patient is suffering from periodic limb movements of sleep (PLMS) or periodic limb movement disorder (PLMD), for which a polysomnograph test is recommended.

B Incorrect. Multiple sleep latency tests are recommended for narcolepsy without cataplexy and idiopathic hypersomnia.

C Incorrect. Maintenance of wakefulness tests are recommended for treatment assessment for narcolepsy, with or without cataplexy and idiopathic hypersomnia.

D–G Incorrect.

References

Kushida CA, Littner MR, Morgenthaler T, et al. Practice parameters for the indications for polysomnography and related procedures: an update for 2005. *Sleep* 2005;**28**(4):499–521.

Littner MR, Kushida CA, Wise M, et al. Practice parameters for clinical use of the multiple sleep latency test and the maintenance of wakefulness test. *Sleep* 2005;**28**(1):113–21.

Disorders of sleep and wakefulness and their treatment

QUESTION EIGHT

A patient recently diagnosed with narcolepsy and treated with a stimulant comes to your office with concerns about attention problems associated with narcolepsy, which he read about on the Internet and which have not been responsive to his treatment so far. Which of the following is true?

A. As a sleep disorder, narcolepsy is usually not associated with cognitive disturbances

B. The cognitive disturbances associated with narcolepsy can be worsened by stimulants

C. Stimulants used to treat narcolepsy can restore cognitive performance

D. Narcolepsy can sometimes lead to cognitive disturbances, but little is known about treating these

Answer to Question Eight

The correct answer is C.

Choice	Peer answers
A. As a sleep disorder, narcolepsy is usually not associated with cognitive disturbances	4%
B. The cognitive disturbances associated with narcolepsy can be worsened by stimulants	13%
C. Stimulants used to treat narcolepsy can restore cognitive performance	70%
D. Narcolepsy can sometimes lead to cognitive disturbances, but little is known about treating these	13%

A and D Incorrect. Individuals with untreated narcolepsy have difficulty sustaining attention, which is associated with inefficient activation in the dorsolateral prefrontal cortex and is indicated by poor performance on an n-back test.

B Incorrect. Stimulants can improve, not worsen, cognitive disturbances associated with narcolepsy.

C Correct. Dopaminergic wake-promoting agents may enable individuals with narcolepsy to sustain activation of the dorsolateral prefrontal cortex, thus improving cognitive performance. For this patient, modafinil, a higher dose of his stimulant, or a different stimulant may successfully treat these symptoms.

References

Stahl SM. *Stahl's essential psychopharmacology*, fourth edition. New York, NY: Cambridge University Press; 2013. (Chapter 11)

QUESTION NINE

A patient started working a night shift as a security guard 1 week ago. At this time, he is most likely to have a disrupted _____ drive while his _____ drive is unaffected.

A. Ultradian. . . circadian

B. Circadian. . .homeostatic

C. Homeostatic. . .ultradian

D. Ultradian. . .homeostatic

E. Circadian. . .ultradian

F. Homeostatic. . .circadian

Answer to Question Nine

The correct answer is B.

Choice	Peer answers
A. Ultradian. . . circadian	2%
B. Circadian. . .homeostatic	65%
C. Homeostatic. . .ultradian	2%
D. Ultradian. . .homeostatic	0%
E. Circadian. . .ultradian	20%
F. Homeostatic. . .circadian	11%

B Correct. Circadian (wake) drive is the result of input such as light, melatonin, and physical activity to the suprachiasmatic nucleus. Homeostatic (sleep) drive increases the longer one is awake without sleep and is associated with an accumulation of the neurotransmitter adenosine. An individual working a night shift is not likely to receive normal light input although (s)he may sleep a normal amount and therefore is likely to have a disrupted circadian drive with an unaffected homeostatic drive.

Over time, however, individuals who do shift work often sleep fewer hours than they would on a normal schedule – but not because they actually need less sleep – and thus their homeostatic drive can build up.

A, C, D, and E Incorrect. Ultradian cycle refers to the cyclical recurrence of the multiple phases of sleep and is most likely unaffected in this normal individual.

F Incorrect.

References

Czeisler CA, Gooley JJ. Sleep and circadian rhythms in humans. *Cold Spring Harb Symp Quant Biol* 2007;**72**:579–97.

Stahl SM. *Stahl's essential psychopharmacology*, fourth edition. New York, NY: Cambridge University Press; 2013. (Chapter 11)

QUESTION TEN

A 24-year-old paramedic frequently works night shifts and is having difficulty staying alert throughout his shift. As part of your recommendations for addressing sleep hygiene, you should advise that he:

A. Avoid caffeine

B. Use caffeine only in the early part of his shift

C. Use caffeine throughout his shift

Answer to Question Ten

The correct answer is B.

Choice	Peer answers
A. Avoid caffeine	9%
B. Use caffeine only in the early part of his shift	87%
C. Use caffeine throughout his shift	4%

A and C Incorrect. Caffeine can actually be a useful tool for dealing with excessive sleepiness in individuals with shift work sleep disorder. However, its use must be timed correctly in order not to induce wakefulness when they need to sleep.

B Correct. Shift workers with performance issues due to sleepiness may consume small amounts of caffeine early in the shift in order to stay alert.

References

Pandi-Perumal SR, Srinivasan V, Maestroni GJ, et al. Melatonin: nature's most versatile biological signal? *FEBS J* 2006;**273**:2813–38.

Schwartz JR, Roth T. Shift work sleep disorder: burden of illness and approaches to management. *Drugs* 2006;**66**:2357–70.

Disorders of sleep and wakefulness and their treatment

QUESTION ELEVEN

A clinician is planning to prescribe eszopiclone for a 34-year-old male patient with insomnia. What is the correct starting dose for this patient?

A. 0.5 mg/night

B. 1 mg/night

C. 2 mg/night

D. 3 mg/night

Answer to Question Eleven

The correct answer is B.

Choice	Peer answers
A. 0.5 mg/night	19%
B. 1 mg/night	64%
C. 2 mg/night	15%
D. 3 mg/night	2%

A   Incorrect (0.5 mg/night).

B   Correct. In 2014 the FDA reduced the recommended starting dose of eszopiclone from 2 mg/night to 1 mg/night for both men and women. This is because, in some patients, eszopiclone blood levels may be high enough the next morning to cause impairment in activities that require alertness, including driving. In 2013, the FDA issued new dosing requirements for zolpidem due to the risk of next-morning impairment. However, the label change applied only to dosing in women (5 mg IR, 6.25 mg XR).

C   Incorrect (2 mg/night). Prior to the revised dosing requirements in 2014, the recommended dose range for eszopiclone was 2–3 mg/night; however, that is no longer the case.

D   Incorrect (3 mg/night). Prior to the revised dosing requirements in 2014, the recommended dose range for eszopiclone was 2–3 mg/night; however, that is no longer the case.

References

Stahl SM. *Stahl's essential psychopharmacology, the prescriber's guide*, fifth edition. New York, NY: Cambridge University Press; 2014.

QUESTION TWELVE

A 28-year-old woman with chronic insomnia is hoping to find an effective treatment but is reluctant to try anything that might cause dependence. Her clinician is considering prescribing suvorexant, which acts as an antagonist at orexin receptors. Specifically, what type of orexin antagonists may be effective for treating patients with sleep–wake disorders?

A. Single orexin receptor antagonists selective for orexin 1 receptors

B. Single orexin receptor antagonists selective for orexin 2 receptors

C. Dual orexin receptor antagonists that block both orexin 1 and 2 receptors

D. A and B

E. B and C

F. A and C

G. A, B, and C

Answer to Question Twelve

The correct answer is E.

Choice	Peer answers
A. Single orexin receptor antagonists selective for orexin 1 receptors	16%
B. Single orexin receptor antagonists selective for orexin 2 receptors	11%
C. Dual orexin receptor antagonists that block both orexin 1 and 2 receptors	33%
D. A and B	4%
E. B and C	27%
F. A and C	2%
G. A, B, and C	7%

A Incorrect. Orexin serves to stabilize and promote wakefulness. Its postsynaptic actions are mediated by two receptors: orexin 1 and orexin 2. Orexin 1 receptors are highly expressed in the locus coeruleus, where noradrenergic neurons originate, and are thought to play only a supplementary role in sleep/wake regulation. Consistent with this, preclinical trials with single orexin receptor antagonists for orexin 1 receptors have not demonstrated an effect on sleep.

B Partially correct. Orexin 2 receptors are highly expressed in the tuberomammillary nucleus, where histaminergic neurons originate. It is believed that the effect of orexin on wakefulness is largely mediated by activation of the TMN histaminergic neurons that express orexin 2 receptors. Presumably, orexin 2 receptors therefore play a pivotal role in sleep/wake regulation. Consistent with this, there are promising preclinical results of single orexin receptor antagonists for orexin 2 receptors.

C Partially correct. Dual orexin receptor antagonists, such as suvorexant, have evidence of efficacy in the treatment of insomnia.

D Incorrect (A and B).

E Correct (B and C).

F Incorrect (A and C).

G Incorrect (A, B, and C).

References

Stahl SM. *Stahl's essential psychopharmacology*, fourth edition. New York, NY: Cambridge University Press; 2013.

QUESTION THIRTEEN

The suprachiasmatic nucleus, or "circadian pacemaker," is influenced by activity, light, and which one of the following neurotransmitters?

A. Acetylcholine

B. Melatonin

C. Norepinephrine

D. Serotonin

Answer to Question Thirteen

The correct answer is B.

Choice	Peer answers
A. Acetylcholine	2%
B. Melatonin	96%
C. Norepinephrine	0%
D. Serotonin	2%

A Incorrect. Acetylcholine is formed in cholinergic neurons and is primarily involved in cognitive functioning. It does not have a prominent role in regulation of circadian rhythms.

B Correct. Melatonin is secreted by the pineal gland and mainly acts in the suprachiasmatic nucleus to regulate circadian rhythms.

C Incorrect. Norepinephrine is involved in many functions, including sleep. However, it does not have a primary role in regulating the suprachiasmatic nucleus.

D Incorrect. Serotonin, like norepinephrine, is involved in many functions, including sleep. It does not, however, play a prominent role in regulating the suprachiasmatic nucleus.

References

Arendt J. Melatonin and the pineal gland: influence on mammalian seasonal and circadian physiology. *Rev Reproduction* 1998;**3**:13–22.

Stahl SM. *Stahl's essential psychopharmacology*, fourth edition. New York, NY: Cambridge University Press; 2013. (Chapter 11)

Chapter peer comparison

For the Disorders of sleep and wakefulness section, the correct answer was selected 66% of the time.

Disorders of sleep and wakefulness and their treatment

8 ATTENTION DEFICIT HYPERACTIVITY DISORDER (ADHD) AND ITS TREATMENT

QUESTION ONE

A 15-year-old with inattentive-type attention deficit hyperactivity disorder has a hard time staying focused on the task at hand, has trouble organizing her work, and relies heavily on her mother to follow through with her homework. Problem solving is one of the hardest tasks for her. Her difficulty with sustained attention could be related to aberrant activation in the:

A. Dorsolateral prefrontal cortex

B. Prefrontal motor cortex

C. Orbital frontal cortex

D. Supplementary motor cortex

Answer to Question One

The correct answer is A.

Choice	Peer answers
A. Dorsolateral prefrontal cortex	84%
B. Prefrontal motor cortex	11%
C. Orbital frontal cortex	5%
D. Supplementary motor cortex	0%

A **Correct. Sustained attention** is hypothetically modulated by the cortico-striatal-thalamic-cortical loop involving the **dorsolateral prefrontal cortex** (DLPFC). Inefficient activation of the DLPFC can lead to problems following through or finishing tasks, disorganization, and trouble sustaining mental effort; the patient exhibits all of these symptoms. The dorsal **anterior cingulate cortex** is important in regulating **selective attention**, and is associated with behaviors such as losing things, being distracted, and making careless mistakes. This area is certainly also inefficient in this patient.

B Incorrect. The **prefrontal motor cortex** hypothetically modulates behaviors such as fidgeting, leaving one's seat, running/climbing, having trouble being quiet.

C Incorrect. The **orbital frontal cortex** on the other hand regulates impulsivity, which includes symptoms such as talking excessively, blurting things out, and interrupting others.

D Incorrect. Finally, the **supplementary motor area** is implicated in planning motor actions; thus this brain area would be more involved in hyperactive symptoms.

References

Arnsten AF. Fundamentals of attention-deficit/hyperactivity disorder: circuits and pathways. *J Clin Psychiatry* 2006;**67** (Suppl 8):7–12.

Stahl SM. *Stahl's essential psychopharmacology*, fourth edition. New York, NY: Cambridge University Press; 2013. (Chapter 12)

Stahl SM, Mignon L. *Stahl's illustrated attention deficit hyperactivity disorder.* New York, NY: Cambridge University Press; 2009. (Chapter 1)

Attention deficit hyperactivity disorder (ADHD) and its treatment

QUESTION TWO

Which of the following is true regarding cortical brain development in children with ADHD compared to healthy controls?

A. The pattern (i.e., order) of cortical maturation is different

B. The timing of cortical maturation is different

C. The pattern and timing of cortical maturation are different

D. Neither the pattern nor the timing of cortical maturation are different

Answer to Question Two

The correct answer is B.

Choice	Peer answers
A. The pattern (i.e., order) of cortical maturation is different	7%
B. The timing of cortical maturation is different	42%
C. The pattern and timing of cortical maturation are different	47%
D. Neither the pattern nor the timing of cortical maturation are different	4%

Attention deficit hyperactivity disorder, or ADHD, is a neurodevelopmental disorder characterized by inattentive, hyperactive, and/or impulsive symptoms. Some posit that ADHD results from a delay in brain maturation, while others believe that it reflects complete deviation from typical brain development. Neuroimaging has been used to evaluate cortical maturation in children with ADHD compared to typically developing controls, specifically by comparing the age of attaining peak cortical thickness in children with and without ADHD.

A Incorrect. Research shows that the pattern of cortical maturation is similar for children with and without ADHD. Specifically, the primary sensory and motor areas attain peak cortical thickness earlier in development than do high-order association areas such as the dorsolateral prefrontal cortex.

B Correct. There are differences in the timing of cortical maturation between children with and without ADHD that are apparent as early as age 7. That is, cortical maturation in children with ADHD seems to lag behind that of healthy children. In fact, the median age by which 50% of the cortical points achieve peak thickness is delayed by 3 years in children with ADHD. Delay is most prominent in the superior and dorsolateral prefrontal regions, which are particularly important for control of attention and planning.

Interestingly, there is one brain region in which children with ADHD achieve peak cortical thickness earlier than typically developing controls: the primary motor cortex.

C and D Incorrect.

References

Shaw P, Eckstrand K, Sharp W, et al. Attention-deficit/hyperactivity disorder is characterized by a delay in cortical maturation. *PNAS* 2007;**104**(49):19649–54.

QUESTION THREE

A clinician is considering treatment options for a 26-year-old man with ADHD who has a history of alcohol and marijuana abuse. Which of the following accurately explains the effects of different stimulant formulations on neuronal firing?

A. Pulsatile stimulation amplifies undesirable phasic dopamine (DA) and norepinephrine (NE) firing, which can lead to euphoria and abuse

B. Immediate-release stimulants lead to tonic firing, which can lead to euphoria and abuse

C. Tonic firing is the result of rapid receptor occupancy and fast onset of action as seen with extended release formulations

D. Extended release stimulants result in phasic stimulation of NE and DA signals, but this does not lead to euphoria and abuse

Answer to Question Three

The correct answer is A.

Choice	Peer answers
A. Pulsatile stimulation amplifies undesirable phasic DA and NE firing, which can lead to euphoria and abuse	58%
B. Immediate-release stimulants lead to tonic firing, which can lead to euphoria and abuse	15%
C. Tonic firing is the result of rapid receptor occupancy and fast onset of action as seen with extended release formulations	1%
D. Extended release stimulants result in phasic stimulation of NE and DA signals, but this does not lead to euphoria and abuse	26%

A Correct. **Pulsatile** delivery of stimulants can cause a **frequent and rapid** increase in NE and DA, and this amplifies **phasic firing**. Phasic firing is hypothetically associated with **reward, feelings of euphoria,** and abuse potential.

B Incorrect. **Immediate–release stimulants** rapidly increase DA and NE, thereby especially increasing phasic firing, not tonic firing. Therefore, immediate-release stimulants have a higher risk of abuse.

C and D Incorrect. Extended release formulations of stimulants lead to a **gradual and sustained** increase in NE and DA, thus enhancing **tonic firing**, which is hypothetically linked to the **therapeutic effects** of stimulants. They are amplifying tonic NE and DA signals, which are thought to be low in ADHD. The extended release formulations **occupy the NE transporter** in the prefrontal cortex with slow enough onset and for long enough to enhance tonic NE and DA signaling; however, they do not block DA transporters fast or long enough in the nucleus accumbens to increase phasic signaling, thus reducing abuse potential.

References

Schatzberg AF, Nemeroff CB. *Textbook of psychopharmacology*, fourth edition. Washington, DC: American Psychiatric Publishing, Inc.; 2009. (Chapter 43)

Stahl SM. *Stahl's essential psychopharmacology*, fourth edition. New York, NY: Cambridge University Press; 2013. (Chapter 12)

QUESTION FOUR

Scarlet, a 25-year-old bartender, was diagnosed with ADHD at age 10. She has been on and off medication since then; first on immediate-release methylphenidate, then on the methylphenidate patch. She has experimented with illicit drugs during her late adolescence and is still a heavy drinker. After a few years of self-medication with alcohol and cigarettes, she is seeking medical attention again. You decide to put her on 80 mg/day of atomoxetine, one of the non-stimulant medications effective in ADHD. Why does atomoxetine lack abuse potential?

A. It decreases norepinephrine levels in the nucleus accumbens, but not in the prefrontal cortex

B. It increases dopamine levels in the prefrontal cortex but not in the nucleus accumbens

C. It modulates serotonin levels in the raphe nucleus

D. It increases dopamine in the striatum and anterior cingulate cortex

Answer to Question Four

The correct answer is B.

Choice	Peer answers
A. It decreases norepinephrine levels in the nucleus accumbens, but not in the prefrontal cortex	16%
B. It increases dopamine levels in the prefrontal cortex but not in the nucleus accumbens	74%
C. It modulates serotonin levels in the raphe nucleus	8%
D. It increases dopamine in the striatum and anterior cingulate cortex	2%

Atomoxetine is a selective norepinephrine reuptake inhibitor (NET inhibitor).

A Incorrect. In the nucleus accumbens there are only a few NE neurons and NE transporters. **Inhibiting NET in the nucleus accumbens** will not lead to an increase in NE or DA.

B Correct. The prefrontal cortex lacks high concentrations of DAT, so in this brain region, DA gets inactivated by NET. Therefore, **inhibiting NET in the prefrontal cortex** increases both DA and NE. As only a few NET exist in the nucleus accumbens, atomoxetine does not induce an increase in DA and NE in the nucleus accumbens, the reward center of the brain, thus atomoxetine does not have abuse potential.

C Incorrect. Atomoxetine does not modulate serotonin levels.

D Incorrect. The striatum and the anterior cingulate cortex are not brain areas involved in reward.

References

Schatzberg AF, Nemeroff CB. *Textbook of psychopharmacology*, fourth edition. Washington, DC: American Psychiatric Publishing, Inc.; 2009. (Chapter 43)

Stahl SM. *Stahl's essential psychopharmacology*, fourth edition. New York, NY: Cambridge University Press; 2013. (Chapter 12)

QUESTION FIVE

Patrick, a 15-year-old high school student, has trouble finishing his math tests within the allotted time because he gets easily distracted. In his English literature class, his grades are poor because of careless spelling mistakes. His pediatrician suggests testing his selective attention using the _____ to see if the _____ is aberrantly activated on an fMRI[*].

A. Stroop Task; orbital frontal cortex

B. N-back Test; prefrontal motor cortex

C. Stroop Task; anterior cingulate cortex

D. N-back Test; dorsolateral prefrontal cortex

[*]this is a hypothetical question, as imaging techniques, while important research tools, cannot, to this date, be used for diagnostic purposes

Attention deficit hyperactivity disorder (ADHD) and its treatment

Answer to Question Five

The correct answer is C.

Choice	Peer answers
A. Stroop Task; orbital frontal cortex	11%
B. N-back Test; prefrontal motor cortex	2%
C. Stroop Task; anterior cingulate cortex	55%
D. N-back Test; dorsolateral prefrontal cortex	32%

A, B, and D Incorrect. The **N–back test** is used to look at the activation of the **dorsolateral prefrontal cortex** in order to assess **sustained attention and problem solving**. The **orbital frontal cortex** is hypothetically involved in **impulsivity** and not attention, and the **prefrontal motor cortex** is hypothetically linked to **hyperactivity**, so both choices are not adequate in this case.

C Correct. The **Stroop task** is used to test **selective attention**. In the Stroop task, the participant is shown words that are written in a different **color**. The goal is to name the color in which the word is written, not read the word itself. For example, if the word "blue" is written in "red," then the correct answer is "red." The **anterior cingulate cortex** is involved in this type of task, and will activate when the participant does this task. Inefficient activation of the anterior cingulate cortex is related to symptoms such as paying little attention to details, making careless mistakes, not listening, and getting distracted; these are all symptoms that Patrick is experiencing.

References

Stahl SM. *Stahl's essential psychopharmacology*, fourth edition. New York, NY: Cambridge University Press; 2013. (Chapter 12)

QUESTION SIX

A 15–year–old patient with ADHD has a rare mutation in the gene for the dopamine transporter (DAT). In deciding which treatment to initiate for this patient's ADHD, you know it will be important to avoid treatments that depend on normally functioning DAT. Which of the following drugs are transported into neurons via the dopamine transporter?

A. Amphetamine

B. Atomoxetine

C. Methylphenidate

D. A and B

E. None of the above

Answer to Question Six

The correct answer is A.

Choice	Peer answers
A. Amphetamine	56%
B. Atomoxetine	9%
C. Methylphenidate	11%
D. A and B	10%
E. None of the above	13%

A Correct. Amphetamine blocks DAT and the norepinephrine transporter (NET) by binding at the same site that the monoamines bind. Thus, amphetamine is a competitive inhibitor and pseudosubstrate for DAT and NET, such that (at least at high doses) amphetamine is actually transported into the presynaptic DA terminal.

B Incorrect. Atomoxetine is an inhibitor of NET (binding at a site distinct from where monoamines bind) but does not have actions at DAT.

C Incorrect. Methylphenidate blocks DAT and NET by binding at sites distinct from where monoamines bind (i.e., allosterically). Thus, it stops the transporters so that no monoamine (or methylphenidate) is transported into the neurons. This is similar to how most antidepressant reuptake inhibitors work.

D and E Incorrect.

References

Schatzberg AF, Nemeroff CB. *Textbook of psychopharmacology*, fourth edition. Washington, DC: American Psychiatric Publishing, Inc.; 2009. (Chapter 43)

Stahl SM. *Stahl's essential psychopharmacology*, fourth edition. New York, NY: Cambridge University Press; 2013. (Chapter 12)

Stahl SM. *Stahl's essential psychopharmacology, the prescriber's guide*, fifth edition. New York, NY: Cambridge University Press; 2014.

QUESTION SEVEN

Peter, a 35–year–old stockbroker, has been advised by his supervisor to come and see you, the company mental health consultant. His supervisor is complaining that he often comes late to appointments, is inappropriately fidgety, interrupts people during meetings, has been offensive towards coworkers, and has been known to party excessively on weeknights. Peter asserts that he is just fine; he has a lot of projects on his mind and is simply standing up for himself when speaking with others. He likes to go out in the evenings to unwind. Recognizing probable ADHD you are interviewing both the patient and his work buddy, who is a longtime friend. How would you start your questions?

A. Compared to his parents, how often does the patient. . .

B. Compared to other people his age, how often does the patient. . .

C. Compared to his childhood, how often does the patient. . .

D. Compared to his children, how often does the patient. . .

Attention deficit hyperactivity disorder (ADHD) and its treatment

Answer to Question Seven

The correct answer is B.

Choice	Peer answers
A. Compared to his parents, how often does the patient...	1%
B. Compared to other people his age, how often does the patient...	84%
C. Compared to his childhood, how often does the patient...	16%
D. Compared to his children, how often does the patient...	0%

The symptoms of ADHD can **present differently** in patients at **different ages**. While **hyperactivity** is a main symptom in children for example, this will most likely translate into **internal restlessness** in adults.

A and D Incorrect. While ADHD has a strong genetic component, it is not advised to ask him first to compare himself to either his children or his parents. An accurate family history however would be beneficial.

B Correct. When trying to diagnose this adult patient with ADHD, it is preferable to **first** ask him to **compare his behavior** to that of **other adults his age**, as this will give a better idea of the severity of his symptoms at this time.

C Incorrect. While it is important to obtain a medical history, the patient might not have the best recollection and might not be the best judge of his behaviors as a child.

References
Stahl SM. *Stahl's essential psychopharmacology*, fourth edition. New York, NY: Cambridge University Press; 2013. (Chapter 12)

QUESTION EIGHT

A 28-year-old patient with generalized anxiety disorder has been treated successfully with paroxetine for 3 years. He also has a childhood history of ADHD but is not currently being treated for it. In addition, he has a history of stimulant abuse, but has been clean for several years. He presents now stating that he is having significant work impairment due to inattention and disorganization and is in danger of losing his job. Full evaluation reveals that he does meet criteria for current ADHD. Because of his history of substance abuse, atomoxetine is chosen as a treatment. What pharmacokinetic interaction, if any, would you expect between atomoxetine and paroxetine?

A. Atomoxetine is an inducer of CYP450 2D6 and paroxetine is metabolized by CYP450 2D6, so the dose of paroxetine should be increased

B. Paroxetine is an inducer of CYP450 2D6 and atomoxetine is metabolized by CYP450 2D6, so the dose of atomoxetine should be increased

C. Atomoxetine is an inhibitor of CYP450 2D6 and paroxetine is metabolized by CYP450 2D6, so the dose of paroxetine should be decreased

D. Paroxetine is an inhibitor of CYP450 2D6 and atomoxetine is metabolized by CYP450 2D6, so the dose of atomoxetine should be decreased

Answer to Question Eight

The correct answer is D.

Choice	Peer answers
A. Atomoxetine is an inducer of CYP450 2D6 and paroxetine is metabolized by CYP450 2D6, so the dose of paroxetine should be increased	8%
B. Paroxetine is an inducer of CYP450 2D6 and atomoxetine is metabolized by CYP450 2D6, so the dose of atomoxetine should be increased	12%
C. Atomoxetine is an inhibitor of CYP450 2D6 and paroxetine is metabolized by CYP450 2D6, so the dose of paroxetine should be decreased	17%
D. Paroxetine is an inhibitor of CYP450 2D6 and atomoxetine is metabolized by CYP450 2D6, so the dose of atomoxetine should be decreased	64%

Atomoxetine is **metabolized** by CYP450 2D6, meaning that any drug that **inhibits** CYP450 2D6 will **increase the levels** of atomoxetine. Paroxetine is an inhibitor of CYP450 2D6.

A Incorrect. Atomoxetine is not an inducer of CYP450 2D6.

B Incorrect. Paroxetine is not an inducer of CYP450 2D6.

C Incorrect. Atomoxetine is not an inhibitor of CYP450 2D6.

D Correct. In the **presence of paroxetine**, the dose of **atomoxetine** should be **decreased**.

References

Schatzberg AF, Nemeroff CB. *Textbook of psychopharmacology*, fourth edition. Washington, DC: American Psychiatric Publishing, Inc.; 2009. (Chapter 43)

Stahl SM. *Stahl's essential psychopharmacology*, fourth edition. New York, NY: Cambridge University Press; 2013. (Chapter 12)

Stahl SM. *Stahl's essential psychopharmacology, the prescriber's guide*, fifth edition. New York, NY: Cambridge University Press; 2014.

QUESTION NINE

A 44-year-old patient with newly-diagnosed ADHD has severe liver damage caused by many years of heavy drinking. You know that while most medications used for ADHD should be used with caution or not at all in patients with cardiac impairments, there is only one drug that requires special care when prescribing it to a person with liver impairment. Which drug is it?

A. Lisdexamfetamine

B. D-methylphenidate

C. D,L-methylphenidate

D. Atomoxetine

E. D,L-amphetamine

F. D-amphetamine

Answer to Question Nine

The correct answer is D.

Choice	Peer answers
A. Lisdexamfetamine	13%
B. D-methylphenidate	2%
C. D,L-methylphenidate	3%
D. Atomoxetine	73%
E. D,L-amphetamine	8%
F. D-amphetamine	2%

B and C Incorrect. Methylphenidate is mainly not metabolized by the liver.

D Correct. Atomoxetine needs to be **adjusted** in patients with hepatic impairment. For patients with **moderate** liver impairment, the dose should be **reduced to 50%** of the normal dose. For patients with **severe** liver damage, the drug should be **reduced to 25%** of the normal dose. In addition, atomoxetine itself can rarely cause severe liver damage.

A, E, and F Incorrect. Amphetamine is partially metabolized by the liver, and D-amphetamine is the only stimulant that might need to be used with caution in patients with hepatic impairment; all others are fine to use in this patient.

References

Bangs ME, Jin L, Zhang S, et al. Hepatic events associated with atomoxetine treatment for attention-deficit hyperactivity disorder. *Drug Saf* 2008;**31**(4):345–54.

Schatzberg AF, Nemeroff CB. *Textbook of psychopharmacology*, fourth edition. Washington, DC: American Psychiatric Publishing, Inc.; 2009. (Chapter 43)

Stahl SM. *Stahl's essential psychopharmacology*, fourth edition. New York, NY: Cambridge University Press; 2013. (Chapter 12)

Stahl SM. *Stahl's essential psychopharmacology, the prescriber's guide*, fifth edition. New York, NY: Cambridge University Press; 2014.

QUESTION TEN

A 7-year-old boy has just been diagnosed with ADHD, combined type, and his care provider feels that the best therapeutic choice is a stimulant. Family history is significant for depression and diabetes. The patient's medical history is significant for asthma; physical exam reveals no abnormalities. According to current recommendations, what should be the care provider's next step?

A. Prescribe a stimulant, as no additional tests are indicated for this patient

B. Obtain an electrocardiogram (ECG), as this patient's family history and exam results warrant it

C. Obtain an ECG, as this is mandatory prior to prescribing a stimulant to any child

D. Prescribe a non-stimulant, as a stimulant would not be appropriate for this patient

Answer to Question Ten

The correct answer is A.

Choice	Peer answers
A. Prescribe a stimulant, as no additional tests are indicated for this patient	77%
B. Obtain an electrocardiogram (ECG), as this patient's family history and exam results warrant it	4%
C. Obtain an ECG, as this is mandatory prior to prescribing a stimulant to any child	12%
D. Prescribe a non-stimulant, as a stimulant would not be appropriate for this patient	7%

A Correct. Current recommendations from the American Heart Association (AHA) are that it is reasonable but not mandatory to obtain an electrocardiogram (ECG) prior to prescribing a stimulant to a child. The American Academy of Pediatrics (AAP) does not recommend an ECG prior to starting a stimulant for most children.

B Incorrect. According to recommendations, it is at the physician's discretion whether or not to obtain an ECG; however, in this case there is no evidence of cardiovascular disease in either the family history or patient exam.

C Incorrect. According to AHA and AAP recommendations, treatment with a stimulant should not be withheld because an ECG is not obtained.

D Incorrect. There is no reason why a stimulant would not be a reasonable choice for this patient.

References

American Academy of Pediatrics/American Heart Association. American Academy of Pediatrics/American Heart Association clarification of statement on cardiovascular evaluation and monitoring of children and adolescents with heart disease receiving medications for ADHD. *J Dev Behav Pediatr* 2008;**29**(4):335.

QUESTION ELEVEN

A 24-year-old woman has just been diagnosed with ADHD and is going to begin taking medication. She is adamant about not being put on a medication that "is known to make you an addict and will lead to heroin abuse." Her psychiatrist chooses to prescribe lisdexamfetamine, because it is approved for adults and because it is the only amphetamine to date that may theoretically lack abuse potential. Why is this?

A. Lisdexamfetamine is absorbed intact from the gut and then enzymatically converted to amphetamine in the blood and thus is only slowly absorbed

B. Lisdexamfetamine must be enzymatically converted to amphetamine in the bloodstream to become effective, and thus enters the brain slowly

C. Lisdexamfetamine is packaged with slow-release technology that becomes ineffective with tampering

D. Lisdexamfetamine is packaged with slow-release technology that prevents the "kick" experienced with immediate-release amphetamine

Attention deficit hyperactivity disorder (ADHD) and its treatment

Answer to Question Eleven

The correct answer is A.

Choice	Peer answers
A. Lisdexamfetamine is absorbed intact from the gut and then enzymatically converted to amphetamine in the blood and thus is only slowly absorbed	80%
B. Lisdexamfetamine must be enzymatically converted to amphetamine in the bloodstream to become effective, and thus enters the brain slowly	6%
C. Lisdexamfetamine is packaged with slow-release technology that becomes ineffective with tampering	3%
D. Lisdexamfetamine is packaged with slow-release technology that prevents the "kick" experienced with immediate-release amphetamine	10%

A Correct. Lisdexamfetamine is the prodrug of D–amphetamine. It is only metabolically active once it has been absorbed by the intestinal wall and converted into the active compound D–amphetamine and L–lysine within red blood cells.

B Incorrect.

C and D Incorrect. Lisdexamfetamine is a prodrug and is not packaged with slow-release technology.

References

Dew RE, Kollins SH. Lisdexamfetamine dimesylate: a new option in stimulant treatment for ADHD. *Expert Opin Pharmacother* 2010;**11**(17): 2907–13.

Stahl SM, Mignon L. *Stahl's illustrated attention deficit hyperactivity disorder.* New York, NY: Cambridge University Press; 2009.

QUESTION TWELVE

Rita is a 28-year-old patient with untreated ADHD. You are currently deciding between guanfacine and clonidine as potential treatments for this patient. The selective alpha 2A agonist guanfacine appears to be:

A. Less tolerated than the alpha 2 agonist clonidine

B. Better tolerated than the alpha 2 agonist clonidine

C. Less efficacious than the alpha 2 agonist clonidine

D. More efficacious than the alpha 2 agonist clonidine

Attention deficit hyperactivity disorder (ADHD) and its treatment

Answer to Question Twelve

The correct answer is B.

Choice	Peer answers
A. Less tolerated than the alpha 2 agonist clonidine	6%
B. Better tolerated than the alpha 2 agonist clonidine	77%
C. Less efficacious than the alpha 2 agonist clonidine	6%
D. More efficacious than the alpha 2 agonist clonidine	10%

There are two direct-acting agonists for alpha 2 receptors used to treat ADHD, guanfacine and clonidine. Guanfacine is relatively more selective for alpha 2A receptors than for other subtypes, whereas clonidine binds to alpha 2A, alpha 2B, and alpha 2C receptors. Clonidine also has actions on imidazoline receptors, which is thought to be responsible for some of clonidine's sedating and hypotensive actions.

A Incorrect. Although the actions of clonidine at alpha 2A receptors exhibit therapeutic potential for ADHD, its actions at other receptors may increase side effects. By contrast, guanfacine is 15–60 times more selective for alpha 2A receptors than for α2B and α2C receptors. Additionally, guanfacine is 10 times weaker than clonidine at inducing sedation and lowering blood pressure. Thus, guanfacine is better tolerated than clonidine.

B Correct. Guanfacine is better tolerated than clonidine.

C Incorrect. Guanfacine is 25 times more potent in enhancing prefrontal cortical function. Thus, it can be said that guanfacine exhibits therapeutic efficacy with a reduced side-effect profile compared to clonidine.

D Incorrect. There are no head-to-head comparisons to establish that guanfacine has superior efficacy to clonidine in ADHD.

References

Stahl SM. *Stahl's essential psychopharmacology*, fourth edition. New York, NY: Cambridge University Press; 2013. (Chapter 12)

Stahl SM. *Stahl's essential psychopharmacology, the prescriber's guide*, fifth edition. New York, NY: Cambridge University Press; 2014.

QUESTION THIRTEEN

A 44-year-old man was diagnosed with ADHD-inattentive subtype in college but has not taken medication for the last several years. He is seeking treatment now because of declining work performance following a promotion 7 months ago. Specifically, he complains of difficulty finishing papers and staying focused during meetings and fears that his boss is losing confidence in him. Assessment confirms a diagnosis of ADHD-inattentive subtype. After 2 months treatment on a therapeutic dose of a long-acting stimulant, he states that his focus, sustained attention, and distractibility are much better, but that he still can't get organized and that it takes him longer to complete tasks than it should. At this point, would it be appropriate to raise the dose of the stimulant to try to address his residual symptoms?

A. Yes

B. No

Answer to Question Thirteen

The correct answer is B.

Choice	Peer answers
A. Yes	53%
B. No	47%

A Incorrect. Dose–response studies of stimulant medications suggest that the optimal dose varies across individuals and depends somewhat on the domain of function. Specifically, higher doses may lead to greater improvement of some domains (e.g., vigilance, attention) but not executive function (e.g., planning, cognitive flexibility, inhibitory control).

B Correct. If medication dose is high enough to substantially diminish symptoms of inattention and distractibility, then executive function needs to be addressed independently and will not likely respond to higher medication dosing.

References

Pietrzak RH, Mollica CM, Maruff P, Snyder PJ. Cognitive effects of immediate-release methylphenidate in children with attention-deficit/hyperactivity disorder. *Neurosci Biobehav Rev* 2006;**30**:1225–45.

Swanson J, Baler RD, Volkow ND, et al. Understanding the effects of stimulant medications on cognition in individuals with attention-deficit hyperactivity disorder: a decade of progress. *Neuropsychopharmacology* 2011;**36**:207–26.

Chapter peer comparison

For the Attention deficit hyperactivity disorder (ADHD) section, the correct answer was selected 67% of the time.

9 DEMENTIA AND COGNITIVE FUNCTION AND ITS TREATMENT

QUESTION ONE

Mary, a 79-year-old patient, is brought to your office by her daughter, who reports that her mother has been exhibiting several concerning symptoms over the past year. Comprehensive questioning reveals that her symptoms are: trouble remembering familiar things, such as telephone numbers commonly dialed; not recognizing some close family members who visit often; moodiness; and difficulty performing writing tasks. Although not definitive, these symptoms are most likely indicative of which type of dementia?

A. Alzheimer's disease

B. Dementia with Lewy bodies

C. Huntington's disease

D. Frontotemporal dementia

Answer to Question One

The correct answer is A.

Choice	Peer answers
A. Alzheimer's disease	89%
B. Dementia with Lewy bodies	2%
C. Huntington's disease	0%
D. Frontotemporal dementia	10%

Differential diagnosis of dementias can be difficult, as all are characterized by the core symptom of memory impairment. However, it may be possible to distinguish dementias clinically through other presenting symptoms.

A Correct. In addition to memory impairment, Alzheimer's disease consists of deficits in language (aphasia), motor function (apraxia), recognition (agnosia), or executive functioning, all of which this patient exhibits. Definitive diagnosis, however, is not possible until autopsy.

B Incorrect. Dementia with Lewy bodies is often accompanied by extrapyramidal symptoms, which this patient does not have.

C Incorrect. Huntington's disease is associated with spasmodic movements and incoordination, which are also absent in this patient.

D Incorrect. In frontotemporal dementia, patients often are disinhibited and may be extremely talkative, symptoms that are also not part of this patient's presentation.

References

Schatzberg AF, Nemeroff CB. *Textbook of psychopharmacology*, fourth edition. Washington, DC: American Psychiatric Publishing, Inc.; 2009. (Chapter 48)

Stahl SM. *Stahl's essential psychopharmacology*, fourth edition. New York, NY: Cambridge University Press; 2013. (Chapter 13)

QUESTION TWO

A young man who is pre-med and has a family history of Alzheimer's disease is interested in learning more about the brain regions involved in memory and the development of Alzheimer's disease. You describe the pathways of acetylcholine, an important neurotransmitter involved in dementia. As part of your explanation, you tell him that major cholinergic projections stem from the _____ to the _____, which are believed to be involved in memory.

A. Basal forebrain; nucleus accumbens

B. Basal forebrain; prefrontal cortex

C. Striatum; hypothalamus

D. Striatum; prefrontal cortex

Answer to Question Two

The correct answer is B.

Choice	Peer answers
A. Basal forebrain; nucleus accumbens	7%
B. Basal forebrain; prefrontal cortex	59%
C. Striatum; hypothalamus	15%
D. Striatum; prefrontal cortex	16%

A, C, and D Incorrect.

B Correct. Acetylcholine is an important neurotransmitter, and is thought to be involved in memory. Major acetylcholine neurotransmitter projections originating in the basal forebrain project to the prefrontal cortex, hippocampus, and amygdala.

References

Schatzberg AF, Nemeroff CB. *Textbook of psychopharmacology*, fourth edition. Washington, DC: American Psychiatric Publishing, Inc.; 2009. (Chapter 48)

Stahl SM. *Stahl's essential psychopharmacology*, fourth edition. New York, NY: Cambridge University Press; 2013. (Chapter 13)

Woolf NJ, Butcher LL. Cholinergic systems mediate action from movement to higher consciousness. *Behav Brain Res* 2011;**221**(2):488–98.

QUESTION THREE

A young woman brings her 72-year-old mother for an appointment because she is concerned that her mother may have Alzheimer's disease. The mother does not feel that anything is wrong, but her daughter states that she has seemed somewhat depressed and forgetful lately. Data have shown that:

A. Depression is often comorbid with Alzheimer's disease

B. Depression may increase the risk of developing Alzheimer's disease

C. Depression may be a prodromal symptom of Alzheimer's disease

D. All of the above

E. None of the above

Answer to Question Three

The correct answer is D.

Choice	Peer answers
A. Depression is often comorbid with Alzheimer's disease	2%
B. Depression may increase the risk of developing Alzheimer's disease	2%
C. Depression may be a prodromal symptom of Alzheimer's disease	6%
D. All of the above	88%
E. None of the above	2%

A   Partially correct. Mood symptoms can occur as part of Alzheimer's disease and in fact are typically the first notable symptom (often manifested as apathy rather than sadness). In addition, depression is a common comorbid illness in patients with Alzheimer's disease.

B   Partially correct. Depression has been hypothesized to be a possible risk factor for Alzheimer's disease.

C   Partially correct. Depression has been hypothesized to be a possible prodromal symptom of Alzheimer's disease, with some evidence suggesting that it may exacerbate the progression of Alzheimer's pathology.

D   Correct (all of the above).

E   Incorrect (none of the above).

References

Barnes DE, Yaffe K, Byers AL, et al. Midlife vs late-life depressive symptoms and risk of dementia: differential effects for Alzheimer disease and vascular dementia. *Arch Gen Psychiatry* 2012;**69**(5):493–8.

Pomara N, Bruno D, Sarreal AS, et al. Lower CSF amyloid beta peptides and higher F2-isoprostanes in cognitively intact elderly individuals with major depressive disorder. *Am J Psychiatry* 2012;**169**:523–30.

QUESTION FOUR

A 68-year-old patient with an early diagnosis of Alzheimer's disease is put on a cholinesterase inhibitor in hopes of improving his cognitive function. This patient has been a chain smoker for over 40 years and refuses to give up the habit. Which of the following medications would *not* be appropriate for this patient, given his smoking habit?

A. Donepezil

B. Galantamine

C. Rivastigmine

D. None of these medications should be prescribed to a patient who smokes

E. There are no contraindications due to smoking for these medications

Answer to Question Four

The correct answer is E.

Choice	Peer answers
A. Donepezil	0%
B. Galantamine	22%
C. Rivastigmine	4%
D. None of these medications should be prescribed to a patient who smokes	4%
E. There are no contraindications due to smoking for these medications	71%

E Correct. One can potentially choose any cholinesterase inhibitor as a first-line treatment, since specific contraindications due to smoking do not presently appear in the literature.

A Incorrect. Donepezil, a reversible, long-acting selective inhibitor of acetylcholinesterase (AChE), may be a good choice, resulting in mainly transient gastrointestinal side effects.

B Incorrect. Galantamine has a dual mechanism of action: AChE inhibition and positive allosteric modulation (PAM) of nicotinic cholinergic receptors. This may be a good choice for this patient.

C Incorrect. Rivastigmine, delivered both orally and via a transdermal formulation, has similar safety and efficacy as donepezil. The oral formulation may result in more gastrointestinal side effects than donepezil, owing to its pharmacokinetic profile and inhibition of both AChE and butyrylcholinesterase (BuChE) in the periphery.

D Incorrect.

References
Stahl SM. *Stahl's essential psychopharmacology, the prescriber's guide*, fifth edition. New York, NY: Cambridge University Press; 2014.

Stahl SM. *Stahl's essential psychopharmacology*, fourth edition. New York, NY: Cambridge University Press; 2013. (Chapter 13)

QUESTION FIVE

John, a 73-year-old mid-stage Alzheimer's patient, has been on donepezil, 10 mg/day for approximately 8 months to aid in improving his cognitive functioning. His wife has begun to notice a loss of effectiveness over the past month, and they present today to determine a new course of action. You decide to augment John's donepezil with 5 mg/day of memantine. Which of the following properties of memantine may be useful in treating Alzheimer's disease?

A. Serotonin 3 (5HT3) antagonism

B. Sigma antagonism

C. *N*-methyl-D-aspartate (NMDA) antagonism at the PCP site

D. NMDA antagonism at the magnesium site

Answer to Question Five

The correct answer is D.

Choice	Peer answers
A. Serotonin 3 (5HT3) antagonism	6%
B. Sigma antagonism	0%
C. *N*-methyl-D-aspartate (NMDA) antagonism at the PCP site	27%
D. NMDA antagonism at the magnesium site	67%

A and B Incorrect. Memantine possesses weak 5HT3 antagonist properties and sigma antagonist properties, but it is currently unclear if these contribute to its benefit in Alzheimer's disease.

C Incorrect. Memantine is an NMDA antagonist, but it does not bind at the PCP site.

D Correct. Memantine is an NMDA antagonist that binds to the magnesium site. It works as an uncompetitive open channel NDMA receptor antagonist (i.e., low–moderate affinity, voltage dependence, fast-blocking/unblocking kinetics). Memantine is quickly reversible if phasic bursts of glutamate occur, but is able to block tonic glutamate release from having negative downstream effects. This hypothetically stops the excessive glutamate from interfering with the resting glutamate neuron's physiological activity and thus improving memory.

References

Kotermanski SE, Johnson JW. Mg2+ imparts NMDA receptor subtype selectivity to the Alzheimer's drug memantine. *J Neurosci* 2009;**29**(9): 2774–9.

Schatzberg AF, Nemeroff CB. *Textbook of psychopharmacology*, fourth edition. Washington, DC: American Psychiatric Publishing, Inc.; 2009. (Chapter 57)

Stahl SM. *Stahl's essential psychopharmacology*, fourth edition. New York, NY: Cambridge University Press; 2013. (Chapter 13)

QUESTION SIX

Ruth, a 71-year-old patient with dementia who is taking a choli-nesterase inhibitor, has been exhibiting psychiatric symptoms, including extreme agitation and aggression toward her two daughters who help care for her. Which of the following medications might be tried first to alleviate these presenting symptoms?

A. Citalopram, 20 mg/day

B. Galantamine, 8 mg/twice daily

C. Risperidone, 0.5 mg/day

D. Selegiline, 8 mg/day

Answer to Question Six

The correct answer is A.

Choice	Peer answers
A. Citalopram, 20 mg/day	53%
B. Galantamine, 8 mg/twice daily	2%
C. Risperidone, 0.5 mg/day	45%
D. Selegiline, 8 mg/day	0%

Patients with dementia generally experience behavioral and emotional symptoms as well as cognitive symptoms. Specifically treating agitation and aggression in dementia may be controversial. If possible, managing reversible precipitants of agitation should be attempted first: pain, nicotine withdrawal, medication side effects, undiagnosed medical and neurological illnesses and provocative environments.

A Correct. First-line treatment of agitation and aggression in dementia is generally a selective serotonin reuptake inhibitor (SSRI) or serotonin-norepinephrine reuptake inhibitor (SNRI); thus, citalopram would be an appropriate choice for this patient. The maximum recommended dose of citalopram in the elderly is 20 mg/day.

B Incorrect. When utilizing medications, cholinesterase inhibitors are often considered first-line, but may work better as preventative treatment rather than once symptoms have emerged. This patient is already taking one of these agents.

C Incorrect. There is a black box warning about increased risk of cerebrovascular events and death in elderly patients with dementia who use antipsychotics. Thus, this is not the best choice of those presented and should generally not be used first-line. However, if an atypical antipsychotic were to be administered, risperidone is often preferred, and at low doses.

D Incorrect. Second-line treatments that may help avoid turning to atypical antipsychotics include beta blockers, valproate, gabapentin, pregabalin, and selegiline.

References

Ballard C, Creese B, Corbett A, Aarsland D. Atypical antipsychotics for the treatment of behavioral and psychological symptoms in dementia, with a particular focus on longer term outcomes and mortality. *Expert Opin Drug Saf* 2011;**10**(1):35–43.

Ballard C, Corbett A, Chitramohan R, Aarsland D. Management of agitation and aggression associated with Alzheimer's disease: controversies and possible solutions. *Curr Opin Psychiatry* 2009;**22**(6):532–40.

QUESTION SEVEN

Sam, a 65-year-old patient, is in your office today for a consultation. He admits that he has had a significant lack of interest in golfing, one of his favorite past-times; he is frustrated that it has become seemingly more difficult to swing the club. In addition, he notes that he recently become increasingly agitated when other church parishioners sit in the seat that he prefers during the church service and has even verbally lashed out at them. With this information, how might you best describe Sam's symptoms?

A. Early stages of Alzheimer's disease, focusing on mood changes

B. Depression-executive dysfunction

C. Amnestic mild cognitive impairment

D. Natural aging/elderly disposition symptoms

Answer to Question Seven

The correct answer is B.

Choice	Peer answers
A. Early stages of Alzheimer's disease, focusing on mood changes	22%
B. Depression-executive dysfunction	73%
C. Amnestic mild cognitive impairment	0%
D. Natural aging/elderly disposition symptoms	6%

A Incorrect. Early stages of Alzheimer's may be difficult to diagnose and distinguish from depression–executive dysfunction at this point, but cognitive impairment is not quite apparent. In addition, he is well aware of his own symptoms, which is frequently not the case with Alzheimer's disease.

B Correct. Late-onset depression may be a dysfunction of prefrontal cortico-striatal-thalamic-cortical (CSTC) circuits in relation to executive dysfunction. This may be termed depression–executive dysfunction, or DED, and is characterized by psychomotor retard-ation, reduced interest in activities, impaired insight, and pro-nounced behavioral disability. Often times an episode of depression may be confused with dementia in the elderly.

C Incorrect. Amnestic mild cognitive impairment (MCI) is defined as a memory impairment compared to age-matched peers with normal cognitive function in other domains (no aphasia, apraxia, agnosia, or executive dysfunction) and no functional evidence of actual demen-tia. Since this patient is having problems with apraxia and agitation, this is likely not the correct diagnosis.

D Incorrect. Natural aging would likely not include agitation and aggression, as described here.

References

Alexopoulos GS, Kiosses DN, Heo M, Murphy CF, Shanmugham B, Gunning-Dixon F. Executive dysfunction and the course of geriatric depression. *Biol Psychiatry* 2005;**58**(3):204–10.

Schatzberg AF, Nemeroff CB. *Textbook of psychopharmacology*, fourth edition. Washington, DC: American Psychiatric Publishing, Inc.; 2009. (Chapter 48)

Stahl SM. *Stahl's essential psychopharmacology*, fourth edition. New York, NY: Cambridge University Press; 2013. (Chapter 13)

QUESTION EIGHT

A 79-year-old man presents to your office with his wife. She lists significant medical history, such as chronic renal failure, mild cirrhosis, arrhythmia, and a recent diagnosis of moderately severe Alzheimer's disease by their family physician. Which of the following medications for Alzheimer's disease has a "do not use" warning for patients with renal and hepatic impairment?

A. Donepezil

B. Rivastigmine

C. Memantine

D. Galantamine

Answer to Question Eight

The correct answer is D.

Choice	Peer answers
A. Donepezil	18%
B. Rivastigmine	14%
C. Memantine	26%
D. Galantamine	42%

A Incorrect. Donepezil, a cholinesterase inhibitor, could potentially be given to this patient to aid in treatment of Alzheimer's, though little data has been gathered on its effects in regard to renal and hepatic impairment. Cardiac patients should use this drug with caution due to reports of syncopal episodes.

B Incorrect. Rivastigmine, a cholinesterase inhibitor, appears as though it could be useful in this situation, as it can be used in patients with renal or hepatic impairment; caution should be exercised in cardiac patients due to potential syncopal episodes.

C Incorrect. Memantine, an NMDA receptor antagonist, would be useful in this case due to its indication of approval for treatment of moderate to severe dementia, with which this patient has been diagnosed, although the label indicates a lowered dose for use in severe renal impairment. However, there is not likely to be a problem for hepatic or cardiac impaired patients.

D Correct. Galantamine has a "do not use" warning in patients with renal and hepatic impairment, as well as a caution warning when used in cardiac impaired patients. Furthermore, galantamine, a cholinesterase inhibitor, is often prescribed as one of the first-line treatments for early stage Alzheimer's, rather than moderately severe cases.

References

Schatzberg AF, Nemeroff CB. *Textbook of psychopharmacology*, fourth edition. Washington, DC: American Psychiatric Publishing, Inc.; 2009. (Chapter 48)

Stahl SM. *Stahl's essential psychopharmacology*, fourth edition. New York, NY: Cambridge University Press; 2013. (Chapter 13)

QUESTION NINE

A 65-year-old woman is concerned that her husband is exhibiting some symptoms suggestive of Alzheimer's disease. She is extremely anxious and wants a definitive diagnosis. Which of the following is true regarding the current application of biomarkers for the early detection and differential diagnosis of Alzheimer's disease?

A. There are currently no identified biomarkers that can predict progression to dementia

B. Use of biomarkers in Alzheimer's disease is currently recommended solely for research purposes

C. Use of biomarkers in Alzheimer's disease is just now being recommended for clinical practice

Dementia and cognitive function and its treatment

Answer to Question Nine

The correct answer is B.

Choice	Peer answers
A. There are currently no identified biomarkers that can predict progression to dementia	12%
B. Use of biomarkers in Alzheimer's disease is currently recommended solely for research purposes	70%
C. Use of biomarkers in Alzheimer's disease is just now being recommended for clinical practice	18%

One difficulty in the diagnosis and early treatment of Alzheimer's disease is that diagnostic criteria require both clinical evidence and post-mortem identification of plaques and tangles. As the clinical manifestation of Alzheimer's disease likely occurs years after the initial deposition of beta amyloid, when disease course is probably still modifiable, in vivo detection of Alzheimer pathology is critical for the early detection and management of Alzheimer's disease. Over the past decade, there have been numerous developments in the detection of Alzheimer pathology in vivo. Biomarkers for Alzheimer's disease include cerebrospinal fluid (CSF) measures of beta amyloid and tau, magnetic resonance imaging (MRI) of brain atrophy, and visualization of beta amyloid and glucose metabolism using special tracers coupled with positron emission tomography (PET). Use of these biomarkers has been shown to predict those who are likely to progress from asymptomatic phases and mild cognitive impairment to full-blown dementia.

B Correct. The National Institute on Aging-Alzheimer's Association workgroup recently published revised diagnostic guidelines that utilize these biomarkers for the early detection of Alzheimer pathology and differential diagnosis of Alzheimer's disease. Although the use of biomarkers for Alzheimer's disease is currently recommended solely for research and clinical trial applications, there is great hope that these biomarkers will become clinically relevant in the near future.

A and C Incorrect.

References
Cummings JL. Biomarkers in Alzheimer's disease drug development. *Alzheimer's and Dementia* 2011,**7**:e13–44.

McKhann GM, Knopman DS, Chertkow H, et al. The diagnosis of dementia due to Alzheimer's disease: recommendations from the

National Institute on Aging-Alzheimer's Association workgroups on diagnostic guidelines for Alzheimer's disease. *Alzheimer's and Dementia* 2011;**7**:263–9.

Sperling RA, Aisen PS, Beckett LA, et al. Toward defining the pre-clinical stages of Alzheimer's disease: recommendations from the National Institute on Aging-Alzheimer's Association workgroups on diagnostic guidelines for Alzheimer's disease. *Alzheimer's and Dementia* 2011;**7**:280–92.

QUESTION TEN

An 87-year-old patient with mild cognitive impairment is suspected of being in the early, prodromal stage of Alzheimer's disease. Although currently for research purposes, which biomarker evidence would support a diagnosis of Alzheimer's disease?

A. Decreased cerebrospinal fluid (CSF) levels of amyloid beta

B. Decreased levels of brain amyloid beta on positron emission tomography (PET) scans

C. Both of the above

D. Neither of the above

Answer to Question Ten

The correct answer is A.

Choice	Peer answers
A. Decreased cerebrospinal fluid (CSF) levels of amyloid beta	40%
B. Decreased levels of brain amyloid beta on positron emission tomography (PET) scans	2%
C. Both of the above	24%
D. Neither of the above	34%

A Correct. During the presymptomatic stage of Alzheimer's disease, A beta peptides are slowly and relentlessly deposited into the brain rather than eliminated via the CSF, plasma, and liver. CSF levels of A beta are therefore low and can be used as a biomarker.

B Incorrect. Levels of brain amyloid beta can be detected with PET scans using radioactive neuroimaging tracers that bind to the fibrillar form of amyloid and thus label mature neuritic plaques. In normal controls, amyloid PET imaging shows the absence of amyloid. However, individuals who are cognitively normal may have moderate accumulation of amyloid; these individuals are likely in the presymptomatic first stage of Alzheimer's disease. In the final stage of Alzheimer's disease, when full-blown dementia is clinically evident, a large accumulation of brain amyloid can readily be seen.

C and D Incorrect.

References
Stahl SM. *Stahl's essential psychopharmacology*, fourth edition. New York, NY: Cambridge University Press; 2013. (Chapter 13)

QUESTION ELEVEN

William is a 77-year-old patient with mid- to late-stage Alzheimer's disease (AD). His cognitive impairment has drastically worsened over the past month. The patient's family is concerned that William's rapidly deteriorating cognitive and physical functioning may be due to his medication (donepezil 10 mg/day) no longer working. The treating clinician feels that AD may not be the primary cause of William's recent deterioration. Which comorbid illness most commonly goes undetected in patients with moderate to severe dementia?

A. Bacteriuria

B. Dehydration

C. Hypothyroidism

Answer to Question Eleven

The correct answer is A.

Choice	Peer answers
A. Bacteriuria	66%
B. Dehydration	20%
C. Hypothyroidism	14%

A Correct. Nearly 40% of individuals with dementia may be suffering from an undetected but modifiable illness. Bacteriuria is the most common undiagnosed illness in patients suffering from dementia, and it can lead to incontinence and increased agitation.

B Incorrect. Although untreated dehydration has been found in 3% of individuals with dementia, it is not the most common undetected comorbid illness.

C Incorrect. Although untreated hypothyroidism has been found in 1–3% of individuals with dementia, it is not the most common undetected comorbid illness.

References
Hodgson NA, Gitlin LN, Winter L, et al. Undiagnosed illness and neuropsychiatric behaviors in community residing older adults with dementia. *Alzheimer Dis Associated Disord* 2011;**25**:109–15.

Chapter peer comparison

For the Dementia and cognitive function and its treatment section, the correct answer was selected 66% of the time.

10 SUBSTANCE USE AND IMPULSIVE COMPULSIVE DISORDERS AND THEIR TREATMENT

QUESTION ONE

Your 16-year-old son is thrilled when he wins the 100-meter dash in an important high school competition. This "natural high" is most likely associated with inducing dopamine release in his meso-limbic pathway and in his:

A. Hypothalamus

B. Amygdala

C. Hippocampus

D. Cerebellum

E. Motor cortex

Answer to Question One

The correct answer is B.

Choice	Peer answers
A. Hypothalamus	14%
B. Amygdala	68%
C. Hippocampus	13%
D. Cerebellum	0%
E. Motor cortex	5%

A, C, D, and E Incorrect.

B Correct. The brain can experience a "natural high" from activities such as athletic or intellectual accomplishments. This occurs when dopamine neurons release dopamine in the mesolimbic pathway, which is sometimes known as the "pleasure center" of the brain, and also in the amygdala, a critical component of the reactive reward system, which conditions reward responses in association with pleasurable activities.

References

Schatzberg AF, Nemeroff CB. *Textbook of psychopharmacology*, fourth edition. Washington, DC: American Psychiatric Publishing, Inc.; 2009. (Chapter 49)

Stahl SM. *Stahl's essential psychopharmacology*, fourth edition. New York, NY: Cambridge University Press; 2013. (Chapter 14)

Stahl SM, Grady MM. *Stahl's illustrated substance use and impulsive disorders*. New York, NY: Cambridge University Press; 2012. (Chapter 2)

Substance use and impulsive compulsive disorders and their treatment

QUESTION TWO

Impulsivity is hypothesized to be related to the _____, while compulsivity is hypothesized to be related to the _____.

A. Amygdala, ventral striatum

B. Ventral striatum, amygdala

C. Dorsal striatum, ventral striatum

D. Ventral striatum, dorsal striatum

Answer to Question Two

The correct answer is D.

Choice	Peer answers
A. Amygdala, ventral striatum	18%
B. Ventral striatum, amygdala	5%
C. Dorsal striatum, ventral striatum	20%
D. Ventral striatum, dorsal striatum	56%

Impulsivity and compulsivity can perhaps be best differentiated by how they both fail to control responses: impulsivity as the inability to stop initiating actions, and compulsivity as the inability to terminate ongoing actions. Impulsivity and compulsivity are hypothetically neurobiological drives that are "bottom-up," with impulsivity coming from the ventral striatum, compulsivity coming from the dorsal striatum, and different areas of prefrontal cortex acting "top-down" to suppress these drives.

A Incorrect. The amygdala is involved in reward conditioning and provides input to the striatum, but it is not directly associated with impulsivity. And the dorsal striatum, not the ventral striatum, is associated with compulsivity.

B Incorrect. Although the ventral striatum is linked to impulsivity, the amygdala is not directly linked to compulsivity.

C Incorrect (dorsal striatum, ventral striatum).

D Correct (ventral striatum, dorsal striatum).

References

Stahl SM. *Stahl's essential psychopharmacology*, fourth edition. New York, NY: Cambridge University Press; 2013. (Chapter 14)

QUESTION THREE

Todd is a 34-year-old man with a 10-year history of alcohol dependence, consuming 4–5 standard drinks a day, every day of the week. Due to some recent health problems, he decided to stop drinking and threw out all the alcohol in his home. Six hours later, he presents at urgent care with tremor, elevated pulse rate, sweating, agitation, and anxiety. Based on his presenting symptoms, does this patient need to be admitted?

A. Yes, inpatient management is necessary

B. No, outpatient management is appropriate for this patient

Answer to Question Three

The correct answer is B.

Choice	Peer answers
A. Yes, inpatient management is necessary	54%
B. No, outpatient management is appropriate for this patient	46%

A percentage of individuals who are alcohol dependent will experience alcohol withdrawal syndrome (AWS). Symptoms, including tremor, elevated pulse rate and blood pressure, sweating, agitation, nervousness, sleeplessness, anxiety, and depression, begin within a few hours of discontinuation of alcohol use and may last a few days to a week. In many cases, AWS resolves without complication and does not require treatment. For some patients, however, intervention is necessary.

A Incorrect. Inpatient management is not necessary for this patient. Situations that *would* require inpatient management would include: (1) if he were experiencing more serious symptoms, such as hallucinations, delirium tremens, psychotic symptoms, or seizures; (2) if he had extremely high alcohol intake; or (3) if he had significant psychiatric symptoms.

B Correct. For patients with mild to moderate AWS, such as this patient, treatment can be on an outpatient basis and should focus on the relief of immediate symptoms, the prevention of complications, and the initiation of rehabilitation. This may involve supportive care and the repletion of nutrient, fluid, or mineral deficiencies (especially vitamin B). Benzodiazepines are commonly used to reduce anxiety, agitation, and autonomic hyperactivity as well as reduce the incidence of delirium tremens and seizures. Long-acting benzodiazepines may allow for a smoother course of withdrawal and less frequent dosing, while short-acting benzodiazepines may be preferred for patients with severe liver disorder. Because benzodiazepines have abuse liability and the potential for interaction with alcohol, alternative options, including carbamazepine, valproate, and topiramate, may be preferred.

References

Soyka M. World Federation of Societies of Biological Psychiatry (WFSBP) guidelines for biological treatment of substance use and related disorders, part 1: alcoholism. *World J Biol Psychiatry* 2008;**9**(1):6–23.

Stahl SM, Grady MM. *Stahl's illustrated substance use and impulsive disorders.* New York, NY: Cambridge University Press; 2012. (Chapter 3)

QUESTION FOUR

A 73-year-old man presents to a new primary care provider for a routine physical exam. During the exam, he is asked some basic screening questions about alcohol use. The patient states that he drinks one mixed drink (containing a single 1-ounce shot) each night. How would you assess this patient's drinking behavior?

A. Low-risk drinking

B. At-risk drinking

C. Alcohol use disorder

Answer to Question Four

The correct answer is A.

Choice	Peer answers
A. Low-risk drinking	85%
B. At-risk drinking	11%
C. Alcohol use disorder	4%

For men aged 65 and older and for women, the recommended drinking limits are no more than three drinks per day and no more than seven drinks per week. For men under the age of 65, the recommended drinking limits are no more than four drinks in one day and no more than 14 drinks in one week. Amounts in excess of these would be considered heavy or at-risk drinking but may not necessarily constitute an alcohol use disorder.

A   Correct. This patient is over age 65 and consumes seven drinks per week (1 drink per night). Therefore, he would be considered to have low-risk drinking behavior.

B   Incorrect. Based on the recommended drinking limits, this patient's drinking behavior does not indicate at-risk drinking or an alcohol use disorder.

C   Incorrect. Based on the recommended drinking limits, this patient's drinking behavior does not indicate at-risk drinking or an alcohol use disorder.

References
National Institute on Alcohol Abuse and Addiction (NIAAA). Available at: http://www.niaaa.nih.gov.

Stahl SM, Grady MM. *Stahl's illustrated substance use and impulsive disorders.* New York, NY: Cambridge University Press; 2012. (Chapter 3)

QUESTION FIVE

A 28-year-old painter presents with a severe drinking problem and you affirm the need for pharmacotherapy. When you suggest naltrexone, the curious artist would like to know how this will help. Which might you use as part of your explanation?

A. Naltrexone blocks mu-opioid receptors to reduce the euphoria you might normally experience with heavy drinking

B. Naltrexone blocks metabotropic glutamate receptors (mGluR) to reduce the euphoria you might normally experience with heavy drinking

C. Naltrexone stimulates mu-opioid receptors to reduce the euphoria you might normally experience with heavy drinking

D. Naltrexone stimulates mGluR receptors to reduce the euphoria you might normally experience with heavy drinking

Answer to Question Five

The correct answer is A.

Choice	Peer answers
A. Naltrexone blocks mu-opioid receptors to reduce the euphoria you might normally experience with heavy drinking	96%
B. Naltrexone blocks metabotropic glutamate receptors (mGluR) to reduce the euphoria you might normally experience with heavy drinking	4%
C. Naltrexone stimulates mu-opioid receptors to reduce the euphoria you might normally experience with heavy drinking	0%
D. Naltrexone stimulates mGluR receptors to reduce the euphoria you might normally experience with heavy drinking	0%

A Correct. Blocking mu-opioid receptors might reduce the desire to engage in heavy drinking activity, as doing so will be associated with reduced reward.

B and D Incorrect. Naltrexone is a mu-opioid antagonist. Mu-opioid receptors theoretically contribute to the "high" or euphoria experienced with heavy drinking, similar to their function in opiate abuse.

C Incorrect. Blocking mu-opioid receptors, not stimulating them, is the likely mechanism of naltrexone's efficacy.

References
Stahl SM. *Stahl's essential psychopharmacology*, fourth edition. New York, NY: Cambridge University Press; 2013. (Chapter 14)

Stahl SM, Grady MM. *Stahl's illustrated substance use and impulsive disorders.* New York, NY: Cambridge University Press; 2012. (Chapter 3)

QUESTION SIX

You have been seeing a 39-year-old accountant for several years, and she has recently disclosed her 10-year prescription opiate addiction to you. She is a quite functional addict, but continues seeking opiates to avoid withdrawal effects. Which of the following might you tell her about her potential for recovery?

A. Opioid receptors can readapt to normal but need a reduction in the amount of opiate exposure over time in order to do so

B. Opioid receptors cannot readapt to normal after severe addiction but can reorganize to nearly full functionality with the aid of permanent pharmacotherapy

Answer to Question Six

The correct answer is A.

Choice	Peer answers
A. Opioid receptors can readapt to normal but need a reduction in the amount of opiate exposure over time in order to do so	91%
B. Opioid receptors cannot readapt to normal after severe addiction but can reorganize to nearly full functionality with the aid of permanent pharmacotherapy	9%

A Correct. The brain's elasticity allows for opioid receptors to readapt to normal after some time of abstinence from drug intake. This may be difficult to tolerate, so reinstituting another opiate, such as methadone, or a partial mu-opiate agonist, such as buprenorphine (in combination with naloxone), may assist the detoxification process.

B Incorrect.

References

Stahl SM. *Stahl's essential psychopharmacology*, fourth edition. New York, NY: Cambridge University Press; 2013. (Chapter 14)

Stahl SM, Grady MM. *Stahl's illustrated substance use and impulsive disorders.* New York, NY: Cambridge University Press; 2012. (Chapter 4)

QUESTION SEVEN

A 24-year-old woman with a 6-year history of smoking has decided that she is ready to quit. She is considering nicotine replacement therapy but is concerned that she may just end up dependent on that instead. Which of the available nicotine replacement therapies carries the highest risk of dependence?

A. Gum

B. Lozenge

C. Nasal spray

D. Oral inhaler

E. Transdermal patch

Answer to Question Seven

The correct answer is C.

Choice	Peer answers
A. Gum	12%
B. Lozenge	0%
C. Nasal spray	52%
D. Oral inhaler	21%
E. Transdermal patch	15%

A Incorrect. With the gum, nicotine is absorbed through the mouth; thus, the rate of delivery is slower than with the nasal spray.

B Incorrect. With the lozenge, nicotine is absorbed through the mouth; thus, the rate of delivery is slower than with the nasal spray.

C Correct. The risk of dependence is related to the rate at which a drug enters and leaves the brain. The nasal spray has the fastest nicotine delivery of all nicotine replacement therapies and thus carries the highest risk of dependence.

D Incorrect. Although nicotine is administered with an oral inhaler, it is absorbed in the mouth as opposed to in the lungs.

E Incorrect. The transdermal patch slowly and steadily delivers nicotine (over 16 or 24 hours), reducing the risk of dependence.

References
Physician's desk reference. Montvale, NJ: Thomson PDR; 2010.
Stahl SM, Grady MM. *Stahl's illustrated substance use and impulsive disorders.* New York, NY: Cambridge University Press; 2012. (Chapter 4)

QUESTION EIGHT

Mary is a 33-year-old woman with alcohol use disorder. She consumes several drinks a day nearly every day of the week and has recently had her two children removed from her care. She is motivated to attempt to stop drinking in order to get her children back. She previously attempted to quit cold turkey and on her own, and ended up in the emergency room with severe withdrawal symptoms. Considering these factors, would she be a good candidate for reduced-risk drinking as a goal?

A. Yes

B. No

Answer to Question Eight

The correct answer is B.

Choice	Peer answers
A. Yes	31%
B. No	69%

B Correct. Reduced-risk drinking as a goal is controversial. However, some patients will not agree to abstinence as a goal. For these patients, it can still be beneficial to work with them to reduce their drinking. Reduced-risk drinking may be a better goal for patients with less severe problem drinking, including at-risk drinkers. The strategy for achieving reduced-risk drinking for patients with alcohol use disorder involves agreeing on a plan. Give patients a choice in the goal if possible – this allows them to take part in decisions affecting their lives and also gives them more responsibility for the outcome. Some sample guidelines for reduced risk drinking include the "three As": avoid having more than one drink in one hour; avoid drinking patterns (same people, same places, same time of day), and avoid drinking to deal with problems.

Contraindications for reduced-risk drinking (as opposed to abstinence) include: existing conditions that would be exacerbated by alcohol, use of disulfiram or other agents contraindicated with alcohol, history of failed attempts with reduced-risk drinking, pregnancy or breastfeeding, and a history of severe alcohol withdrawal symptoms. For patients who should pursue abstinence but refuse, one may try to have them agree to a trial period of abstinence and a trial period of reduced-risk drinking; it can be beneficial to use a written contract.

A Incorrect. Because this patient has a history of severe alcohol withdrawal symptoms, she would not be a good candidate for reduced-risk drinking as a goal.

References

Ambrogne JA. Reduced-risk drinking as a treatment goal: what clinicians need to know. *J Subst Abuse Treatment* 2002;**22**(1):45–53.

Stahl SM. *Stahl's essential psychopharmacology*, fourth edition. New York, NY: Cambridge University Press; 2013. (Chapter 14)

Stahl SM, Grady MM. *Stahl's illustrated substance use and impulsive disorders.* New York, NY: Cambridge University Press; 2012. (Chapter 3)

QUESTION NINE

A 23-year-old college student with a history of illicit substance abuse recently tried "bath salts" as a cheap alternative high that won't be detectable in standard drug toxicology screens. A recent study indicates that relative to methamphetamine, the bath salts component methylenedioxypyrovalerone (MDPV) is likely:

A. 10× less addictive

B. Equally addictive

C. 10× more addictive

Answer to Question Nine

The correct answer is C.

Choice	Peer answers
A. 10× less addictive	2%
B. Equally addictive	25%
C. 10× more addictive	73%

C Correct. Animal research suggests that MDPV, one of the components that can be found in bath salts, has a substantially greater addictive potential than methamphetamine. One study in particular demonstrated that, while rats will press a lever 60 times for a single 0.05 mg/kg dose of methamphetamine, they will press a lever 600 times for a single 0.05 mg/kg dose of MDPV.

A and B Incorrect.

References

Aarde SM, Huang PK, Creehan KM, et al. The novel recreational drug 3,4-methylenedioxypyrovalerone (MDPV) is a potent psychomotor stimulant: self-administration and locomotor activity in rats. *Neuropharmacology* 2013;**71**:130–40.

Baumann MH, Partilla JS, Lehner KR. Psychoactive "bath salts": Not so soothing. *Eur J Pharmacol* 2013;**698**:1–5.

Dybdal-Hargreaves NF, Holder ND, Ottoson PE, et al. Mephedrone: Public health risk, mechanisms of action, and behavioral effects. *Eur J Pharmacol* 2013;**714**:32–40.

Eshleman AJ, Wolfrum KM, Hatfield MG, et al. Substituted methcathinones differ in transporter and receptor interactions. *Biochem Pharmacol* 2013;**85**:1803–15.

QUESTION TEN

Peter is a 17-year-old student who has been using spice (synthetic cannabinoid) over the past year. Synthetic cannabinoids such as spice may be associated with an increased risk of psychosis compared to natural marijuana because they:

A. Do not contain cannabidiol

B. Are full rather than partial agonists

C. A and B

D. Neither A nor B

Answer to Question Ten

The correct answer is C.

Choice	Peer answers
A. Do not contain cannabidiol	0%
B. Are full rather than partial agonists	35%
C. A and B	55%
D. Neither A nor B	10%

A Partially correct. Spice use may cause recurrence or exacerbation of preexisting psychotic symptoms, with studies suggesting a possible threefold increased risk of subsequent psychosis. One factor that may explain why this is seen with spice but not generally with natural marijuana is that natural marijuana contains cannabidiol, which is thought to have antipsychotic properties. In contrast, synthetic cannabinoids do not contain cannabidiol.

B Partially correct. Unlike natural marijuana, which is a partial agonist at the cannabinoid 1 (CB-1) receptor, synthetic cannabinoids are full agonists at CB-1. Therefore, they can potentially lead to excessive stimulation of the receptor. In addition, synthetic cannabinoids bind to the CB-1 receptor with 800 times greater affinity than natural marijuana.

C Correct (A and B).

D Incorrect (neither A nor B).

References

Loeffler G, Hurst D, Penn A, Yung K. Spice, bath salts, and the U.S. military: the emergence of synthetic cannabinoid receptor agonists and cathinones in the U.S. Armed Forces. *Milit Med* 2012;**177**(9):1041–8.

Seely KA, Lapoint J, Moran JH, Fattore L. Spice drugs are more than harmless herbal blends: a review of the pharmacology and toxicology of synthetic cannabinoids. *Progr Neuropsychopharmacol Biol Psychiatry* 2012; **39**(2):234–43.

Woo TM, Hanley JR. "How high do they look?": identification and treatment of common ingestions in adolescents. *J Pediatr Health Care* 2013;**27**:135–44.

QUESTION ELEVEN

Eddie is a 43-year-old man who has a 22-year-old daughter with a history of cocaine addiction. He recently heard about a novel cocaine vaccine that is being studied and would like to know more about it. In describing the cocaine vaccine, you explain that a cocaine-induced "high" is experienced when:

A. At least 47% of dopamine transporters are occupied by cocaine

B. At least 97% of norepinephrine transporters are occupied by cocaine

C. Both of the above

Answer to Question Eleven

The correct answer is A.

Choice	Peer answers
A. At least 47% of dopamine transporters are occupied by cocaine	49%
B. At least 97% of norepinephrine transporters are occupied by cocaine	6%
C. Both of the above	45%

A Correct. Studies have shown that the "high" associated with cocaine occurs when at least 47% of dopamine transporters in the brain are occupied by cocaine. When the cocaine vaccine is administered, it causes the production of antibodies that then bind to the vaccine. The antibodies produced in response to the vaccine do not cross into the brain; thus, antibody-bound cocaine remains in the periphery and may therefore reduce the percentage of cocaine-occupied dopamine transporters below the 47% threshold needed to induce a high. One potential advantage of the vaccine is that it prevents cocaine from entering the brain without affecting normal dopamine neurotransmission.

B Incorrect. Although cocaine does bind to the norepinephrine transporter, it is the effects at the dopamine transporter that are primarily responsible for the induced high.

C Incorrect (both of the above).

References

Maoz A, Hicks MJ, Vallabhjosula S, et al. Adenovirus capsid-based anti-cocaine vaccine prevents cocaine from binding to the nonhuman primate CNS dopamine transporter. *Neuropsychopharmacology* 2013;**38**:2170–8.

QUESTION TWELVE

A 26-year-old woman develops a dependence on opioids after taking them during her recovery from knee surgery. She attempts to stop using them on her own, but when she does stop or decreases her dose she experiences nausea, muscle aches, sweating, diarrhea, insomnia, and depression. She and her practitioner decide that buprenorphine would be an appropriate treatment strategy. Which of the following is true?

A. The patient should initiate buprenorphine while down-titrating her current opioid

B. The patient should be in a mild withdrawal state prior to initiating buprenorphine

C. The patient should complete withdrawal before beginning buprenorphine treatment

Answer to Question Twelve

The correct answer is B.

Choice	Peer answers
A. The patient should initiate buprenorphine while down-titrating her current opioid	17%
B. The patient should be in a mild withdrawal state prior to initiating buprenorphine	71%
C. The patient should complete withdrawal before beginning buprenorphine treatment	12%

B Correct. Buprenorphine is a partial opioid agonist. It has stronger affinity for the mu-opioid receptor than other opioids, and thus causes immediate withdrawal if not administered when the patient is already in withdrawal. If the patient is already experiencing withdrawal, however, it will relieve those symptoms. Buprenorphine is commonly combined with naloxone in order to reduce its diversion and intravenous abuse.

Stage	Typical dosage	Visits	Goal
Initiation (7 days)	Patient must be in mild withdrawal state before starting Day 1: 8 mg B/ 2 mg N Day 2: add'l 4 mg/ 1 mg up to 16 mg/4 mg Days 3–7: increase in units of 4 mg/ 1 mg until withdrawal symptoms cease; maximum 32 mg/ 8 mg	At least 2 hours observation with initial dose, then 1–2 visits in first week	Achieve lowest dose that eliminates withdrawal symptoms and illicit opioid use
Stabilization (up to 2 months)	Generally range from 8 mg/2 mg up to 24 mg/6 mg	1/week	Eliminate withdrawal symptoms, side effects, and illicit drug use
Maintenance (based on	Dose as determined	Biweekly or monthly	Address lifestyle changes and

(*cont.*)

Stage	Typical dosage	Visits	Goal
patient needs)	during stabilization		social and psychological needs; if desired plan for medically supervised withdrawal

A and C Incorrect.

References

Dodrill CL, Helmer DA, Kosten TR. Prescription pain medication dependence. *Am J Psychiatry* 2011;**168**(5):466–71.

Stahl SM, Grady MM. *Stahl's illustrated substance use and impulsive disorders.* New York, NY: Cambridge University Press; 2012. (Chapter 4)

QUESTION THIRTEEN

A 23-year-old woman has recently been diagnosed with binge eating disorder. Since the age of 16 she has had episodes where she eats far beyond the point of hunger, typically at night and when she is alone. The patient feels very guilty and disgusted with herself about her eating habits; this is reinforced by her family members, who tell her that she is just weak and should have more self control. Is there evidence to support the idea that individuals can develop an addiction to food?

A. Yes

B. No

Answer to Question Thirteen

The correct answer is A.

Choice	Peer answers
A. Yes	94%
B. No	6%

A Correct. Food has powerful reinforcing effects. The neurobiological basis of eating and appetite is linked not just to the hypothalamus, but also to the connections that hypothalamic circuits make to reward pathways. Following food deprivation, any food will activate reward pathways. However, palatable (i.e., high-fat, high-sugar) foods activate reward pathways more reliably and more potently than do unpalatable foods. Even without food deprivation, highly palatable foods will activate the release of endocannabinoids and ghrelin; this is not true of unpalatable foods.

There is also evidence that the neurobiological changes associated with the progression to compulsive drug use may similarly occur in individuals with compulsive eating behaviors. When exposed to food cues, obese individuals exhibit increased activation, compared to lean individuals, in regions that process palatability. In contrast, obese individuals exhibit decreased activation of reward circuits during actual food consumption. This is analogous to cravings and tolerance in patients with substance use disorders.

Of course, not everyone who is obese has an eating compulsion, since obesity is also related to genetics and to lifestyle factors such as exercise, caloric intake, and the specific content of consumed foods. In fact, studies of brain activation in response to images of food can differentiate between individuals with binge eating disorder and overweight controls; in particular, differences in activation have been noted in the right ventral striatum.

B Incorrect.

References

Lutter M, Nestler EJ. Homeostatic and hedonic signals interact in the regulation of food intake. *J Nutr* 2009;**139**(3):629–32.

Monteleone P, Piscitelli F, Scognamiglio P, et al. Hedonic eating is associated with increased peripheral levels of ghrelin and the endocannabinoid 2-arachidonoyl-glycerol in healthy humans: a pilot study. *J Clin Endocrinol Metab* 2012;**97**:E917–24.

Weygandt M, Schaefer A, Schienle A, Haynes JD. Diagnosing different binge-eating disorders based on reward-related brain activation patterns. *Hum Brain Mapping* 2012;**33**:2135–46.

Chapter peer comparison

For the Substance use and impulsive compulsive disorders and their treatment section, the correct answer was selected 70% of the time.

CME: POSTTEST AND CERTIFICATE

Overall peer comparison

For *Stahl's Self-Assessments in Psychiatry: Multiple Choice Questions for Clinicians*, second edition, the correct answer was selected 65% of the time.

Release/expiration dates

Released: May 1, 2015
CME Credit Expires: April 1, 2018

CME Posttest Study Guide

Optional posttests with CME credits are available for a fee (waived for NEI Members). For participant ease, each chapter has its own posttest and certificate. NOTE: the book as a whole is considered a single activity and credits earned must be totaled and submitted as such to other organizations. To receive a certificate of CME credit or participation, complete the chapter posttest and evaluation, available only online at **neiglobal.com/CME** (under "Book"). If a score of 70% or more is attained, you will be able to immediately print your certificate. If you have questions, call 888–535–5600, or email customerservice@neiglobal.com.

*PLEASE NOTE: Posttests can only be submitted online. The posttest questions have been provided below solely as a study tool to prepare for your online submissions. **Faxed/mailed copies of posttests cannot be processed** and will be returned to the sender. If you do not have access to a computer, contact customer service at 888–535–5600.*

Basic neuroscience

1. Agonists cause ligand-gated ion channels to:
   A. Open wider
   B. Open for a longer duration
   C. Open more frequently

2. Communication between human CNS neurons at synapses is?
   A. Chemical
   B. Electrical
   C. Both A and B
   D. Neither A nor B

3. The direct role of transcription factors is to:
   A. Cause neurotransmitter release
   B. Influence gene expression
   C. Synthesize enzymes
   D. Trigger signal transduction cascades

4. N-methyl-D-aspartate (NMDA) receptors are activated by:
   A. Glutamate
   B. Glycine
   C. Depolarization
   D. Glutamate and glycine
   E. Glutamate and depolarization
   F. Glycine and depolarization
   G. Glutamate, glycine, and depolarization

Psychosis and schizophrenia

1. Based on thorough evaluation of a patient and his history, his care provider intends to begin treatment with a conventional antipsychotic but has not selected a particular agent yet. Which of the following is most true about conventional antipsychotics?
   A. They are very similar in therapeutic profile but differ in side-effect profile
   B. They are very similar in both therapeutic and side-effect profile
   C. They differ in therapeutic profile but are similar in side-effect profile
   D. They differ in both therapeutic and side-effect profile

2. A 37-year-old woman with schizophrenia has failed to respond to two sequential adequate trials of antipsychotic monotherapy (first olanzapine, then aripiprazole). Which of the following are evidence-based treatment strategies for a patient in this situation?
   A. High dose of her current monotherapy (aripiprazole)
   B. Augmentation of her current monotherapy with another atypical antipsychotic
   C. Switch to clozapine

3. A 27-year-old male who has been treated with quetiapine for the last 8 weeks is now having his medication changed to aripiprazole. What is the recommended starting dose for aripiprazole?
   A. Low dose
   B. Middle dose
   C. Full dose

4. A 34-year-old man who has been taking a conventional anti-psychotic for 6 years has begun demonstrating extrapyramidal side effects (EPS), and his clinician elects to switch him to an atypical antipsychotic with serotonin 2A antagonism. The majority of atypical antipsychotics:
   A. Have higher affinity for dopamine 2 receptors than for serotonin 2A receptors
   B. Have higher affinity for serotonin 2A receptors than for dopamine 2 receptors

Unipolar depression

1. A 36-year-old man with major depressive disorder has lab work done to assess his levels of inflammatory markers. The results come back indicating elevated levels of tumor necrosis factor-alpha (TNF-alpha) and interleukin 6 (IL-6). Elevated cytokine levels may indirectly lead to:
   A. Excessive glutamate and reduced serotonin
   B. Excessive glutamate and excessive serotonin
   C. Reduced glutamate and reduced serotonin
   D. Reduced glutamate and excessive serotonin

2. A 36-year-old patient has only partially responded to his second monotherapy with a first-line antidepressant. Which of the following has the best evidence of efficacy for augmenting antidepressants in patients with inadequate response?
   A. Adding an atypical antipsychotic
   B. Adding buspirone
   C. Adding a stimulant

3. Margaret is a 42-year-old patient with untreated depression. She is reluctant to begin antidepressant treatment due to concerns about treatment-induced weight gain. Which of the following antidepressant treatments is associated with the greatest risk of weight gain?
   A. Escitalopram
   B. Fluoxetine
   C. Mirtazapine
   D. Vilazodone

4. A 38-year-old patient with depression presents with depressed mood, anhedonia, and loss of energy. These symptoms can be conceptualized as reflecting reduced positive affect and are hypothetically more likely to respond to agents that enhance:
   A. Serotonin and possibly dopamine function
   B. Dopamine and possibly norepinephrine function
   C. Norepinephrine and possibly serotonin function

Bipolar disorder

1. A 28-year-old woman presents with a depressive episode. She has previously been hospitalized and treated for a manic episode but is not currently taking any medication. The agents with the strongest evidence of efficacy in bipolar depression are:
   A. Lamotrigine, lithium, quetiapine
   B. Quetiapine, olanzapine-fluoxetine, lurasidone
   C. Olanzapine-fluoxetine, lurasidone, lamotrigine
   D. Lurasidone, lamotrigine, lithium

2. A 24-year-old woman with no history of psychiatric symptoms presents with a major depressive episode and is prescribed an antidepressant. She quickly experiences improved mood and exhibits symptoms suggestive of hypomania. Recommendations from the International Society for Bipolar Disorders (ISBD) state that the patient's antidepressant should be:
   A. Discontinued
   B. Maintained, but ONLY IF a mood stabilizer is added

3. A 24-year-old man with bipolar disorder is being initiated on lithium, with monitoring of his levels until a therapeutic serum concentration is achieved. Once the patient is stabilized, how often should his serum lithium levels be monitored (excluding one-off situations such as dose or illness change)?
   A. Every 2 to 3 months
   B. Every 6 to 12 months
   C. Every 1 to 2 years
   D. Routine monitoring is not necessary

4. Which drugs would theoretically reduce glutamate release by blocking voltage-sensitive sodium channels?
   A. Gabapentin
   B. Levetiracetam
   C. Pregabalin
   D. Valproate

Anxiety disorders

1. A 51-year-old male veteran with chronic PTSD has agreed to begin pharmacotherapy for his debilitating symptoms of arousal and anxiety associated with his experiences in Iraq 2 years ago. Which of the following would be appropriate as first-line treatment?
   A. Paroxetine
   B. Paroxetine or diazepam
   C. Paroxetine, diazepam, or D-cycloserine
   D. Paroxetine, diazepam, D-cycloserine, or quetiapine

2. A 57-year-old man presents with OCD who has not responded to numerous previous trials of serotonergic medications at typical depression doses. Which of the following is true regarding the appropriate dosing of SSRIs in OCD?
   A. Doses are typically lower than those in depression
   B. Doses are typically the same as those in depression
   C. Doses are typically higher than those in depression

3. Which of the following is a strategy currently being investigated for PTSD?
   A. Modulating glutamate neurotransmission during fear conditioning
   B. Modulating glutamate neurotransmission during fear extinction

4. A 31-year-old female assault victim who is brought to the ER appears traumatized from the incident. Which of the following pharmacotherapy options has been theorized as a potential preemptive treatment to the development of PTSD?
   A. N-methyl-D-aspartate (NMDA) agonist such as D-cycloserine
   B. Alpha 2 delta ligand such as pregabalin
   C. Beta adrenergic blocker such as propranolol
   D. Benzodiazepine such as diazepam

Chronic pain

1. A 29-year-old woman has just been diagnosed with major depressive disorder and is being prescribed a selective serotonin reuptake inhibitor (SSRI). In addition to depressed mood, she has been experiencing widespread aches and pains. She asks if the SSRI is likely to alleviate her painful physical symptoms as well as her emotional ones. Which of the following statements is true?
   A. SSRIs may have inconsistent effects on pain because serotonin can both inhibit and facilitate ascending nociceptive signals
   B. SSRIs may worsen pain because serotonin can facilitate but not inhibit ascending nociceptive signals
   C. SSRIs generally alleviate pain because serotonin can inhibit but not facilitate ascending nociceptive signals
   D. SSRIs generally have no effect on pain because serotonin neither facilitates nor inhibits nociceptive signals

2. A 22-year-old woman with pain throughout her body, extreme fatigue, and poor sleep is diagnosed with fibromyalgia. Her care

provider considers prescribing pregabalin, which may alleviate pain by:

A. Binding to the closed conformation of voltage-sensitive sodium channels

B. Binding to the open conformation of voltage-sensitive sodium channels

C. Binding to the closed conformation of voltage-sensitive calcium channels

D. Binding to the open conformation of voltage-sensitive calcium channels

3. A 36-year-old woman has just been diagnosed with fibromyalgia. In addition to her painful physical symptoms, she is experiencing problems with memory and significant difficulty concentrating at work. Which of the following may be most likely to alleviate both her physical pain and her cognitive symptoms?

A. Bupropion

B. Cyclobenzaprine

C. Milnacipran

D. Pregabalin

Sleep/wake disorders

1. Denise is a 32-year-old patient with shift work disorder who reports that she is having difficulty in her job as a pastry chef due to excessive sleepiness during her shift. Which of the following is a potential therapeutic mechanism to promote wakefulness?

A. Inhibit GABA activity

B. Inhibit histamine activity

C. Inhibit orexin activity

2. A 72-year-old woman has been having difficulty sleeping for several weeks, including both difficulty falling asleep and frequent nighttime awakenings. Medical examination rules out an underlying condition contributing to insomnia, and she is not taking any medications that are associated with disrupted sleep. The patient is retired and spends the day caring for her grandchildren, including driving the older ones to school in the morning. Which of the following would be the most appropriate treatment option for this patient?

A. Flurazepam

B. Temazepam

C. Zaleplon

D. Zolpidem CR

CME: posttest and certificate

3. A clinician is planning to prescribe eszopiclone for a 34-year-old male patient with insomnia. What is the correct starting dose for this patient?
   A. 0.5 mg/night
   B. 1 mg/night
   C. 2 mg/night
   D. 3 mg/night

4. What type of orexin antagonists may be effective for treating patients with sleep–wake disorders?
   A. Single orexin receptor antagonists selective for orexin 1 receptors
   B. Single orexin receptor antagonists selective for orexin 2 receptors
   C. Dual orexin receptor antagonists that block both orexin 1 and 2 receptors
   D. A and B
   E. B and C
   F. A and C
   G. A, B, and C

Attention deficit hyperactivity disorder

1. Which of the following is true regarding cortical brain development in children with ADHD compared to healthy controls?
   A. The pattern (i.e., order) of cortical maturation is different
   B. The timing of cortical maturation is different
   C. The pattern and timing of cortical maturation are different
   D. Neither the pattern nor the timing of cortical maturation are different

2. A 44-year-old man is diagnosed with ADHD-inattentive subtype following an assessment that confirms problems with focus, sustained attention, and executive function. After 2 months treatment on a therapeutic dose of a long-acting stimulant, his focus and sustained attention are much better, but he still has trouble with executive function. At this point, would it be appropriate to raise the dose of the stimulant to try to address his residual symptoms?
   A. Yes
   B. No

3. A 25-year-old woman with a history of drug use is diagnosed with ADHD and prescribed atomoxetine. Why does atomoxetine lack abuse potential?
   A. It decreases norepinephrine levels in the nucleus accumbens, but not in the prefrontal cortex

B. It increases dopamine levels in the prefrontal cortex but not in the nucleus accumbens

C. It modulates serotonin levels in the raphe nucleus

D. It increases dopamine in the striatum and anterior cingulate cortex

Dementia and cognitive function

1. Which of the following properties of memantine may be primarily responsible for its therapeutic actions in Alzheimer's disease?
   A. Serotonin 3 (5HT3) antagonism
   B. Sigma antagonism
   C. N-methyl-D-aspartate (NMDA) antagonism at the magnesium site

2. Ruth, a 71-year-old patient with dementia who is taking a cholinesterase inhibitor, has been exhibiting psychiatric symptoms, including extreme agitation and aggression toward her two daughters who help care for her. Which of the following medications might be tried first to alleviate these presenting symptoms?
   A. Citalopram, 20 mg/day
   B. Galantamine, 8 mg/twice daily
   C. Risperidone, 0.5 mg/day
   D. Selegiline, 8 mg/day

3. A 65-year-old woman is concerned that her husband is exhibiting some symptoms suggestive of Alzheimer's disease. She is extremely anxious and wants a definitive diagnosis. Which of the following is true regarding the current application of biomarkers for the early detection and differential diagnosis of Alzheimer's disease?
   A. There are currently no identified biomarkers that can predict progression to dementia
   B. Use of biomarkers in Alzheimer's disease is currently recommended solely for research purposes
   C. Use of biomarkers in Alzheimer's disease is just now being recommended for clinical practice

Substance use and impulsive-compulsive disorders

1. Impulsivity is hypothesized to be related to the _____, while compulsivity is hypothesized to be related to the _____.
   A. Amygdala, ventral striatum
   B. Ventral striatum, amygdala
   C. Dorsal striatum, ventral striatum
   D. Ventral striatum, dorsal striatum

2. Peter is a 17-year-old student who has been using spice (synthetic cannabinoid) over the past year. Synthetic cannabinoids such as spice may be associated with an increased risk of psychosis compared to natural marijuana because they:
   A. Do not contain cannabidiol
   B. Are full rather than partial agonists
   C. A and B
   D. Neither A nor B

3. A 26-year-old woman develops a dependence on opioids after taking them during her recovery from knee surgery. She attempts to stop using them on her own, but when she does stop or decreases her dose she experiences nausea, muscle aches, sweating, diarrhea, insomnia, and depression. She and her practitioner decide that buprenorphine would be an appropriate treatment strategy. Which of the following is true?
   A. The patient should initiate buprenorphine while down-titrating her current opioid
   B. The patient should be in a mild withdrawal state prior to initiating buprenorphine
   C. The patient should complete withdrawal before beginning buprenorphine treatment

4. A 28-year-old painter presents with a severe drinking problem and you prescribe naltrexone. What is the mechanism of naltrexone?
   A. Naltrexone blocks mu-opioid receptors to reduce the euphoria you might normally experience with heavy drinking
   B. Naltrexone blocks metabotropic glutamate receptors (mGluR) to reduce the euphoria you might normally experience with heavy drinking
   C. Naltrexone stimulates mu-opioid receptors to reduce the euphoria you might normally experience with heavy drinking
   D. Naltrexone stimulates mGluR receptors to reduce the euphoria you might normally experience with heavy drinking

CME online posttests and certificates

Optional posttests with CME credits are available for a fee (waived for NEI Members). For participant ease, each chapter has its own posttest and certificate. NOTE: the book as a whole is considered a single activity and credits earned must be totaled and submitted as such to other organizations. To receive a certificate of CME credit or participation, complete the chapter posttest and evaluation, available only online at **neiglobal.com/CME** (under "Book"). If a score of 70% or more is attained, you will be able to immediately print your certificate. If you have questions, call 888–535–5600, or email customerservice@neiglobal.com.

INDEX

Index

Index